Praise for *Unlike the Heart*

'In Nicola Redhouse's *Unlike the Heart*, theoretical questions of psyche and soma are not remote but urgent concerns, intimately bound to her own family's story and the terrible anxiety she experienced after the births of her children. Intelligent, lucid and knowledgeable, the book itself may be said to embody the discipline of neuropsychoanalysis: it combines the narrative of a single patient with insights from the science of the brain.'

Siri Hustvedt

'A vital account of a struggle: resolute, intelligent and endlessly interesting.'

Helen Garner

'In this original, rigorous, poignant yet witty, and personally urgent work, Redhouse puts Freud and his disciples onto the couch – to scrutinise the art, and possibly science, of psychoanalysis, and, even more ambitiously, to find where brain ends and mind begins. This book is a feat of literary and intellectual fireworks.'

Lee Kofman

'Redhouse has corralled the ordinary and extraordinary madness of motherhood, the history of psychoanalysis, the efficacy of antidepressants, the future of neuroscience, and the complexities of her uniquely introspective family to create a kind of perfect memoir – one that enlarges the reader's knowledge and leaves them with questions about their own existence.'

Steven Amsterdam

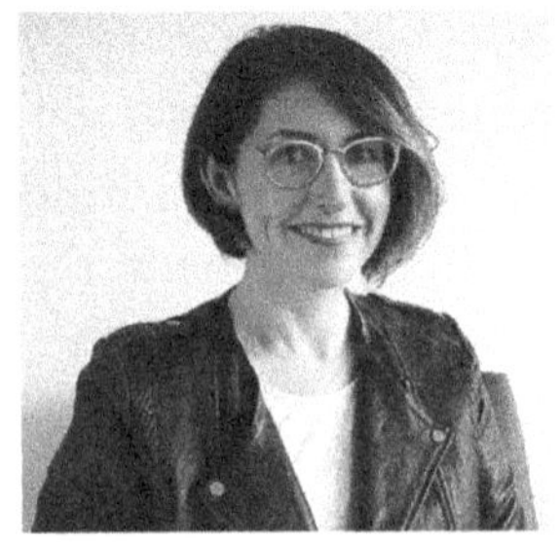

Nicola Redhouse is a writer living in Melbourne, Australia. Her work has been published in the literary journals *Meanjin*, *Island* and *Kill Your Darlings*, and in the anthologies *Best Australian Stories* and *Rebellious Daughters*. She has been working as a book editor since 2005.

UNLIKE THE HEART

A MEMOIR OF BRAIN AND MIND

NICOLA REDHOUSE

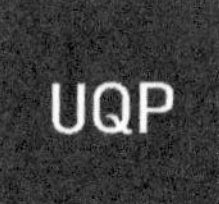

First published 2019 by University of Queensland Press
PO Box 6042, St Lucia, Queensland 4067 Australia

uqp.com.au
uqp@uqp.uq.edu.au

Cover design by Alissa Dinallo
Cover photograph by Tara Moore/Getty Images
Author photograph by JB
Typeset in Bembo Std 11.5/15 pt by Post Pre-press Group, Brisbane
Printed in Australia by McPherson's Printing Group, Melbourne

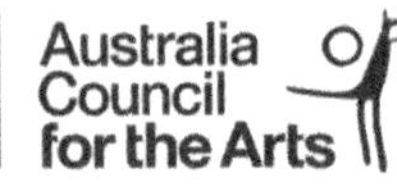

The University of Queensland Press and this project have been assisted by the Australian Government through the Australia Council, its arts funding and advisory body.

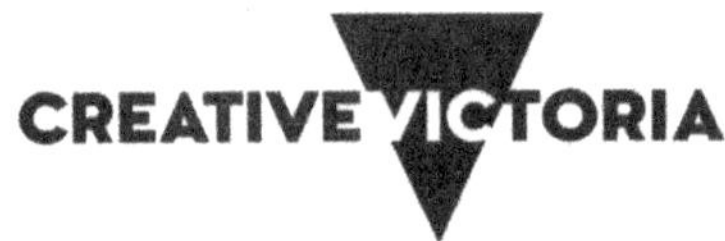

This project is supported by the Victorian Government through Creative Victoria.

A catalogue record for this book is available from the National Library of Australia.

ISBN 978 0 7022 6033 9 (pbk)
ISBN 978 0 7022 6189 3 (pdf)
ISBN 978 0 7022 6190 9 (epub)
ISBN 978 0 7022 6191 6 (kindle)

University of Queensland Press uses papers that are natural, renewable and recyclable products made from wood grown in sustainable forests. The logging and manufacturing processes conform to the environmental regulations of the country of origin.

A woman I don't know
is having a drill drill into her
skull. To get rid of the thing

requires entering the brain.
How to imagine a story
that ends with that ending?

Excerpt from 'Still Life with Antidepressants', Aaron Smith

So long gone had I been
that when I returned
I did not know me, the one

who called – warily, through the trees,
as I approached like a thief or a
          ground mole – *Who is it?*
I saw her whiten in the doorway,
she could have been my cousin.

                              Linda, is that you?
That's what I answered.

From the lintel she took me in, the length
of me, with my one good eye.
Nearing her, I was a worm on end, an indigent.

That was when I knew I had arrived.
The last step is the longest, impassably long, now I will always
be twinned, wanting
to not know returning.

'The Scar', Susan Wheeler

AUTHOR'S NOTE

I want to acknowledge the immense fortune I have in being able to ask the kinds of questions I ask in this book. To be in a position to interrogate my experience is something I can only do because I was able to locate and access the therapeutic help I needed. Mental health access and affordability are catastrophically inadequate in Australia. Currently, while Medicare will cover some of the cost of seeing a psychiatrist for an ongoing period (a medically trained expert in mental illness who may offer medication or a combination of medication and talking therapy, but traditionally the former), it will cover only ten fifty-minute sessions every twelve months with a psychologist (a non-medically trained specialist in mental health treatment). While some psychologists do offer short-term treatments – usually coping strategies and counselling – for a person in emotional crisis looking for a long-term supportive interpersonal therapy that addresses emotional experience deeply (psychodynamic or psychoanalytic therapy), ten funded sessions are nowhere near enough for any kind of valuable work to be done, and is in great disparity to the funding available when mental illness is framed as medical or corporeal, which itself is still inadequate. Without doubt this reflects the strange schism we continue to place between body and mind – as though the two are severable, or one is more real than the other – and the ways we can bring to light robust research findings about each.

I also acknowledge my immense fortune in having a family who has given me their wholehearted support and encouragement to pursue the writing of this book, even when it involves me sifting through and baring aspects of their private lives. The love I have for each of them only deepens as I continue, in my writing and in our lived experiences, to know them more authentically.

I have changed names and identifying details in many cases to maintain the privacy of those who did not ask to have a writer in their midst.

There will be those who encounter this book and turn away from it for the well-worn notion that psychoanalysis is indulgent, navel-gazing. What happens in psychoanalysis can never be about the self on its own; it is always about the self in relation to others. In a world that seems – in the political leaders we elect, in our obsessions with the gloss of celebrity – to increasingly turn away from looking at the ways that power, hatred and mass deceit function in the individual, there is value far beyond the lone person on the couch that comes from the kind of mental work that takes place in psychodynamic therapy.

On the other hand, psychodynamic therapy is not the answer for everyone, and nor can all mental suffering be addressed sufficiently through talking. Nothing in this book is intended to be directive. While I've endeavoured to present the most recent and valid research and theoretical understandings, and have had experts review this work, I am human and quite liable to have misunderstood or introduced mistakes, and new research is constantly underway. Any errors I have made in interpreting, reporting or understanding the research are my own.

PROLOGUE

The second time, I knew what to expect. For three days I had insomnia, dizziness. And then, I felt like myself again. I felt great. I went to my appointment with Dr Parkes, and I had nothing to say. My mind had been swept clean of all the complex feeling I had been wrestling with a few days before. On his chaise longue, with baby Noah on my chest, I slept.

PART 1

1

Before that second time – a few years before – I was seated in a supremely comfortable but ugly feeding chair in my newborn baby's room, sobbing. Not about the chair, although the fleshy symbolism of its pleather folds did provoke some sorrow in me in my vulnerable state.

Crying seemed to be what I did now, even though I felt in love with Reuben, couldn't stop stroking his soft belly, placing my finger in his palm and watching his fingers close around it like an anemone. He was preternaturally strong, and startlingly big: nine pounds ten ounces, a figure that caused my mother, Maxine, to ask repeatedly over the next few weeks if I was sure I hadn't had gestational diabetes. (My mother habitually worried about me developing the illness she had spent her life monitoring in her own body – any time I got very thirsty as a child, she would prick my finger, take blood from me and test my glucose levels.) Reuben latched onto my breast with ease, and sucked strongly and capably, which was lucky for me because I was feeling less than capable.

I hadn't stopped crying since he was born: first, from a truly clichéd maternal joy that I had not expected from myself, and relief that my gruelling labour was finally over. Then, from physical pain – the kind of pain you would expect after delivering a baby that size and needing what felt like several hundred stitches. And finally, from this feeling in me that I couldn't explain or understand or rationalise, but that was like falling at great speed down a black hole. Being un-born.

I wondered if the crying might be a sign of shock; a normal response to my altered life, to my having birthed another human.

Perhaps it was delayed shock at my debilitating pregnancy state. In an epilogue to three months of overwhelming nausea, I had developed a condition that softened the ligaments of my pelvis and caused a sharp ache in my lower back. It destabilised me: I couldn't keep myself upright without a bone-deep gnawing at my pelvis. As the pregnancy progressed, the muscles in my legs, my hips, all trying to hold me together in spite of my loosened joints, cramped and seized. I went to a physio, who taped me back up; I performed repetitive movements on machines that would *engage my core*; over my clothes I wore a strangling velcroed apparatus to keep my ligaments together; under my clothes I wore a thick ribbed elastic sheath to reinforce my growing abdomen; I worked at my glutes with a spiky ball designed to loosen the overcompensating muscles; I iced; I heat-packed; I kept my legs together, as the physio had instructed me, with no trace of irony; I did not lift things. But nothing alleviated the pain.

It had been a lonely time – I was only comfortable lying on my side, so I'd had to surrender not only the things I liked doing but many of the things I was used to taking control of. Cooking, grocery shopping, seeing a friend, getting to work – I could only go places where I could park directly outside or where my husband, Gideon, could drop me, and then I would need to find a seat immediately. I tried using crutches to get about but, lacking a normal centre of gravity, gave up.

Gideon had done most of the baby-preparations that I had hoped to do: the pram-buying, picture-hanging, linen-sorting. I had become entirely dependent on him for anything physical. I'd stopped my work as a book editor a few weeks earlier than I had hoped to, unable to make it up the stairs to my office, or even to sit at my desk anymore. Instead, I lay on the couch at home with the dog, an icepack on my lower back, watching a cat in the neighbouring apartments watch me back. Soon after, on one last hurrah before parenthood, we went to Canberra where friends we had come to visit found a wheelchair I could use and took us around Parliament House. I spent the rest of the time lying on the bed in our extravagant presidential suite feeling little more than the gnawing pain and my own incapacity, and pushing away a growing fear that if the pain did not go after labour I would struggle to look after my baby.

Perhaps all mothers who gave birth to babies Reuben's size cried like this, I now wondered, marvelling at his long legs. I'd had no premonition that he would be a big baby. At my hospital check-ups, where I'd sensed a bureaucratic emphasis on measurement that seemed curiously detached from any purpose – stacks of blood-glucose test strips in the toilet for patient use that were never collected – a midwife had used a measuring tape to ascertain the rudimentary distance from the highest point of my abdomen to the lowest point. This was meant to correlate with the number of weeks' gestation I was at, but at thirty-three weeks it had been four weeks behind what it should have been. Concerned, they'd sent me for a scan. 'He'll be average, about three kilos,' another midwife told me, glooping cold gel around my hardened belly with an ultrasound stick.

But when Reuben was born, the midwives gasped – 'He's nine pounds ten!' one exclaimed, and when I looked at her blankly she translated: '4.35 kilos!' In the year that followed, I would get used to women pulling their lips back into a grimace, hissing out breath or puffing their cheeks when I told them how much he weighed. Not one item of the clothing we had bought for his foray into the world fit: in his first photo he is bursting out of a white terry-towelling onesie, buttons popping.

Or perhaps I was in shock from my labour, which had not been bearable even for moments, as I had hoped. I had blacked out for some of it. 'You're not progressing,' a midwife told me too many times. They had tried to coax progress out of me with the drug Syntocinon, with a student midwife who I began to feel responsible for letting down, so that when she stretched my cervix clumsily and caused me searing pain I couldn't bring myself to cry openly.

And then the real pain had unleashed itself, wild and ruthless. I couldn't find a gap to breathe, and they told me the baby was posterior and my contractions were coming without breaks, and I was still not progressing. I had been lucid, then, in the way one is in a dream, aware of how odd my thoughts were, how loose. I took whatever drugs were on offer: pethidine and gas, anti-emetics. My voice was hoarse – 'I'm being run over by a train!' I screamed at one point, and begged for an epidural. Finally it came, and I had five hours of numbed rest. I drifted in and out of sleep, opening my eyes now and again to a window overlooking a courtyard in the hospital, where a lone poplar tree stood in the half-light of dawn. I found it alien, as though I had never seen a tree.

At 5.50 am a midwife woke me and said it was time to push. I couldn't feel the lower half of my body, so I concentrated on a theoretical idea of pushing instead. They pulled Reuben out with forceps and laid him on my chest. He was extraordinary: solid, alert, with eyes downturned like my mother's, skin slightly jaundiced to make him look olive. *He looks like a Himalayan Sherpa*, I thought to myself, although I later realised I was, in my dream-state, thinking of a beautiful Inuit baby I had once seen in a magazine. Gideon took him to dress him in the too-small onesie, and the medical team descended on my disembodied lower half to put me back together. I was hazy and exhausted, emptied of both the baby and myself. I cried as I stood in the shower of the delivery room and tried to remain upright on my wobbly legs, which were slowly regaining feeling. I cried as I washed away blood – a lot of blood – that had come from me, and that, despite the prenatal classes and all the books, I did not know would come with such ferocity. I cried as I tried to eat a smoked salmon bagel – my request – that my in-laws had brought me, and as a nurse wheeled me to my room, and as I tried to get into my bed, and as I realised I couldn't lift Reuben with the pain I was feeling. I cried when I looked at my perfect baby and when I didn't look at him. And then, when Gideon was sent home for the night, I cried the hardest, so that the woman in the bed next to me was forced to stop her chatter with her visitor – it was her fourth baby, I'd overheard – and ask me if I was all right. 'It's her first,' I heard her tell the visitor, which made me think it might be normal that I was crying so much.

Gideon: dependable, calm, an un-maimed bystander, slightly shocked by his new role as father but whole, bodily intact and able to recognise poplar trees. He had been sent home on account of there not being a bed for him in my tiny shared room, and the implications of that practical fact came crashing down upon me: he was not essential to this new dyad of life. The baby required only me.

The crying hadn't stopped that night either. I couldn't sleep at all in the hospital; even in the snatches of time when Reuben was quiet, I lay crying. I didn't get out of the bed unless it was to go to the toilet, where I was confronted with the way my body now no longer seemed to abide my needs: urine that came when I did not expect it to, and that did not come when I wanted it to. There, in the tiny cubicle I shared with the mother of four, I cried more, feeling my body was irrevocably wounded. Once, I laughed, but it was a laugh of self-reproach: when I saw the toiletry bag I had packed for my hospital stay and remembered I had packed make-up and a hairdryer, as though I had thought I might still be in my same skin, and capable of applying eye shadow in this new life – or caring to. In the mirror I saw not myself but a gaunt replacement, a kind of avatar, strangely younger, paler and with a body I couldn't recognise – a new flat stomach and breasts now swelled so huge they were comical.

My mother had visited that first day, bringing paper bags full of muffins and rye-bread sandwiches and magazines. 'Who delivered him? Which doctor?' she asked, always interested in that kind of detail. But I had no recollection of who had been there or who had handed him to me, only of the feeling of his warm heaviness on me, and I cried. She had come from Sydney and had been staying at a motel near our house as my labour approached, but now returned back to our house with Gideon, who was in his own kind of new-father shock.

In the middle of that first night, in that lonely hospital place in which it is too bright to sleep but too dim to see properly, I'd stared at the light of my phone, my umbilical cord to life before this. Midwives came and went, shifts clocking over, and when the sun rose I phoned Gideon and cried. 'Baby, you'll be fine,' he whispered to me. I held Reuben and cried.

In between the crying, I'd felt an overwhelming affinity with other mothers; a disbelief that I had not realised they had all survived this. I'd wanted to message even my enemies who were mothers, to say: 'I forgive you. Tell me how to survive.' I'd marvelled that I was crying and I had made it this far with smoked salmon bagels and a hospital and a mobile phone and a husband and an epidural, and that so many women did it without any of those middle-class accoutrements.

In all those days at the hospital I hadn't been able to lift Reuben up; when I tried to it felt as though a knife was slicing me in half; I thought of *harakiri*, wondered if I had been disembowelled. I'd had to ring a bell for a nurse every time he cried. Sometimes it took ten minutes for the nurse to arrive, and his and my crying merged together, the two of us lying helplessly in our separate cribs.

When the midwives came, they issued a lot of instructions, but I couldn't take any of them in. It was as though someone had short-wired my brain. The feeding and latching and changing and burping came surprisingly instinctively, but I was also told how to care for myself: how to sit, how to strengthen my pelvic floor, *icepacks for blood-vessel engorgement when your milk comes in*, *warm washers to reduce swelling when your supply is too much*, what medications to take and when, how to lodge a birth certificate, what the scores on the baby's hearing test meant, which genetic diseases they were checking for with the Guthrie heel-prick test.

Registrars and orderlies and doctors and obstetricians and nurses had come by to check how I was healing. They'd pulled the curtain aside, exposing me to whoever was walking past as I tried to coax Reuben onto my breast, my shirtfront wide open. I didn't care. I didn't care about anything anymore but keeping the baby happy, because when he cried it felt like I was being squeezed by the throat. A woman had come to offer to take professional photos of us and, used to having my stitches checked every few minutes, I'd lifted the blanket up to show her, too. We laughed at my awkward mistake, but quickly my laughter had turned to crying, so she left. I'd let Gideon bath and change Reuben, because I was still in too much pain to lift him. I'd also given Gideon the hospital menu to fill out, because I couldn't understand it. I couldn't understand wanting food.

On the third day, they'd sent us home. I walked into the hospital corridor just outside my room, still wearing pyjamas – getting dressed seemed a preposterous show developed by people who didn't know about pain – and felt as if I had landed on a new planet. The gravity of Earth felt different: my body felt both lighter and heavier, with the baby outside of me now but requiring my movement to attend to him. The gnawing in my pelvis had gone, replaced by the pain of stitches.

And then I was home. I had my beautiful, thriving boy and my husband alongside me; family members were bringing pots of soup and tidying the house. None of my parents lived in Melbourne yet, but my mother, father and his partner had all flown in from around Australia in the days before Reuben was born to meet their first grandchild. By the time we'd arrived home from the hospital, though, tensions between them had reached a crescendo and my mother had flown back to Sydney after a blazing row with my father. No one could quite explain to me what had happened, but Maxine was not there when I walked in the door, and I needed her with an intensity I hadn't felt for years. The warm, communal space of my own house felt steely cold to me. I was mobilised to flee a great terror I couldn't name. If I drifted into a half-sleep on the couch, when I woke it was with a dread I could not attach to any specific thing. Why was I so scared?

My crying should have stopped, I was sure. I should have been able to eat, I felt certain. But it hadn't. And I couldn't. I had already lost all my baby weight. I was thinner than before I was pregnant. When I tried to eat my throat closed up and the crying started again.

It was the postbox that had caused me to cry the most. I'd seen it from the living room couch, beyond the front windows, out in the territory of the world that continued to exist despite my collapse, and it had terrified me. Letters and gifts were arriving for Reuben, and I cried and cried and cried, and told Gideon that I would never be able to attend to the post again. I begged him to promise me that he would always manage our correspondences.

Outwardly, I seemed to be doing okay. It turned out I was good at feeding my baby; I was good at holding him. I was good at loving him. And because I was afraid of what all my crying meant, I laughed in between it all. I posted pictures on Facebook. People wanted to visit and, although I had begun to feel panic set in about having only slept a handful of broken hours in a week, I let Gideon co-ordinate their visits, and I moved my mouth and sound came out, and I wore clothes and I seemed like a composite person. People came, bearing gifts, and I tried to behave normally, though I was still in agony, unable to move without wincing, carrying a cushion around with me to place on whichever seat I had to sit on. I opened the gifts aware that I was not feeling the requisite pleasure in them: knitted hats and embossed trinket holders seemed incongruous with the endless human mess of our experience, the spurted milk and poo. The careful effort I had put, during pregnancy, into hand-making pompoms to hang from a mobile in Reuben's room now seemed ludicrous, as though I had been in a state of delusion. All the baby home-deco magazines and blogs now seemed like nothing more than a giant ruse, an attempt to stave off the corporeal truth of this whole endeavour.

I seemed not to be able to stop talking about my labour, and at night it replayed in my mind on a loop. I talked repeatedly about the order of events, but I focused on the parts I thought people would find funny, because somewhere inside me I realised that I needed to balance out all the crying or they would know this was serious: the part where Gideon sucked on the gas and I was so high that I thought the police would come and arrest him; the part where I started making the mooing sound that I had heard other women make; the part where the pethidine kicked in and I thought the sister on duty was wearing flippers instead of shoes.

When they left, I sat in the feeding chair, Reuben quietly suckling away in the dark, my crying and the playlist I had carefully curated when I was still an integrated person the only other sounds in the room.

I rocked him and breathed in his sweet smell, and thought about the kinds of inheritance we can see in our bodies, and of the treacherousness of inheritance. Indeed, some turn of DNA had ricocheted down my maternal line so that my baby boy had the same oceanic, hooded eyes that both I and my mother had. And somewhere in my DNA there was always the possibility that my mother's fear would come true and my endocrines would revolt and diabetes would rear its head. And, of course, I had to wonder what the thin thread that passed from my baby to me to my mother and to her mother, and to all the other branches between and from us, might carry to explain why I was crying so much.

2

There are always wisps of folklore that stick from the story of one's birth. Mine, in a hospital in Johannesburg, in Apartheid South Africa in 1979, were:

I was induced two weeks early because of my mother's diabetes.

I was placed in an incubator for three days so my blood sugar levels could be monitored.

I had my head shaved on one side so a drip could be inserted.

The rest of my hair stuck up like a mohawk.

My feet were turned in from how I had lain in the womb.

I was posterior.

Labour for my mother was unbearable.

'After your father left, when you were a baby and you cried at night I brought you into the bed with me. I was so tired,' my mother told me.

I was nine months old when my father left. My mother was living in a townhouse with me, my older sister, Joni, and a poodle named Cuddles, who would become the third dog my parents adopted and then gave away or lost on the city streets. They had a habit of acquiring dogs either of an unreasonable size for their living quarters or with a pull to freedom that surpassed the lure of a full food bowl.

In that townhouse my parents had entered their mid-twenties, their teenage love in atrophy. Maxine was much too tired for someone so young; shocked by the U-turn of her life. She is still shocked, forty years later; but I've always felt the romantic comedy quality, the impossible synchronicity of plot, that led to their union was an obvious foreboding. My father, Aaron, starred as the tall, skinny young man ambling along the beach during the school summer holidays with his gang of friends, coming upon a group of girls – a flotilla? What is the collective noun for young, hopeful women? – with whom they struck up conversation.

My mother was the one with the dark hair and the heavy-lidded eyes lying on the sand. My mother was the one my father spoke to. She told him the name of her high school. 'Oh, I know a girl who goes there,' he told her, grasping for the only person whose name he had heard who went to that school – a girl he had never met but whom his brother, a maths tutor at that school, had mentioned. 'Maxine,' he said. Obviously, my mother was Maxine.

But it is a story that lacks some vitality of information. The fatefulness of it all takes away their individual agency, makes it inevitable, their actions or feelings irrelevant. Did they fall in lust? It is a very important question, this, for piecing together what came later. It is something hardly any children want to know about their parents – and it is not something I easily want to know – but I need to, to understand something of myself.

My mother was only fifteen, my father seventeen. In photos from the early years of their courtship they are physically matched and give the impression of perfect suitability (a plot point I return to frequently for its callous deceptiveness). They are in school dance photos at first, still black and white, both olive-skinned from tanning with baby oil; my father wears thick black-rimmed glasses and his hair is Beatles-short, my mother's ironed straight and long like the film star Ali MacGraw. Then they are in a Polaroid shot, a saturated sunlight bleaching the colours, my father's hair wild and curly with seventies abandon, now with cigarettes, at restaurant tables, in front of beach umbrellas; in one series, they enjoy a picnic of obscenely large and green pickles in a room that gives the air of a hotel, my father with a linen napkin tucked in front of his open-fronted shirt. They are photos of young courtship, of a couple enjoying having an appetite together. But photos are freeze-frames.

It was the summer of 1968 that day on the beach, and circumstances conspired to put a distance between them. South Africa was fighting communism on the Angola border, and young men like my father were being conscripted. They could either be sent to the country's capital, Pretoria, for boot camp and a year of army service, or they could elect to be called up for three weeks of every year as a commando, for fifteen years. Aaron chose the year of army service. They managed a date during that beach holiday – a chaste affair that my mother told me she can't recall – and then my father had to go to Pretoria. His was not a service of hard labour, of gruelling physicality. He was saved from that by his bad eyesight, posted instead to be a clerk in a drill hall, where his thick bifocals were entirely suited to his paper-stack battles.

A few months into that position, he wrote to my mother (content curiously blank in her retellings; I imagine largely an itemisation of his army meals, knowing how he relishes that sort of detail) and *she knew*: this was going to be *it*. I always feel a pang in my heart at this part. I had a first love, a terrible match for me who I felt certain would be The One, so powerful was the rush of that first significant object of attachment in my adulthood. It took a while for the cloud of my own wishes to dissipate so that I could see the real him. We are doomed never to love our actual love objects, but instead to project over them a mirage of former, infantile fantasy-others, as Freud said.

Six months into his army training, Aaron earned the right to free time, came home and asked my mother out on a date. Maxine told me she can't remember that date, either, other than that Aaron's mother arrived to collect her for it, such were the limitations of my parents' youth. The myopia of her memory, usually razor-sharp, foils the answers I seek.

For Maxine, her attraction to my father was clear: he was on that beach celebrating the end of high school with a posse of male friends. They were bright young things – not wild, not particularly brave, but with enough energy to be almost rebellious in that middle-class milieu. They opposed Apartheid, but had enough of their parents' post-Holocaust fear of authority to stop them doing much more than protesting mildly on university campuses. Maxine knew some of them from around the suburbs, brothers of her friends or family acquaintances, but it was Aaron – tall, intelligent – with whom she felt an immediate affinity. They both came from families that valued education above all else. A *match made in heaven*; a *perfect fit*. Those were her words. But it is not her attraction that is the lacuna in their tale.

Still, if there remained any hesitation on either of their parts about whether they were perfectly suited, it was quickly eclipsed by the discovery that they shared an intellectual passion: psychoanalysis. It was not a fashionable interest – Freud had already begun to fall out of favour in the human sciences, with behaviourism and the likes of BF Skinner infiltrating the approach to psychology. If psychoanalysis used unseeable words to search out the unfindable mind, Skinner, famous for his theories of animals' learned responses, poked a finger at the eyeball to set off a reflex. (He invented the operative conditioning chamber, the Skinner Box, in which an animal could learn to perform an action, like pressing a lever, under observation. He also trained pigeons to play ping-pong.)

Both my parents had gravitated toward understanding the self through looking for what was hidden, what required interpretation. My mother, by then in her final year of high school, had been captivated by something her class was reading at the time – *Hamlet*. She'd already been to an analyst as a child, and felt what it was to release herself from emotional distress through this inexplicable process of talking, but she did not consciously connect what she had experienced in analysis with the spark that *Hamlet* ignited.

The story of the tragic prince was her gateway to thinking about Freudian ideas of unconscious motivations and family dynamics. She took herself off to libraries, discovered a reading of the play by the leading figure of the Freudian movement in South Africa at the time, Wulf Sachs.[1] She couldn't understand how anyone could think of it as just a story about an unhappy man. It was obvious to her Hamlet was tortured by his mind, and his family story was at the heart of it. For Sachs, Hamlet's motivation to avoid the repugnant mission of getting revenge for his father's murder by killing his uncle is explained by the Freudian unconscious, and by Freud's idea that all young men experience unconsciously in childhood a conflict that echoes the Greek story of Oedipus: they love their mothers with such ferocity that they see their fathers as rivals and unconsciously fantasise about killing them to take their place. For Sachs, the troubled prince Hamlet was guided by a 'repressed inhibitory force against the desired act of revenge'. Unbeknown even to himself, he did not want to avenge his father. Hamlet was a classical neurotic, in Freudian terms. What's more, for Sachs, the play, as with any work of art, was an expression of the playwright's own unconscious conflicts, clues of which could be found in Shakespeare's own struggles, among them that he had lost his father shortly before writing it, and years before writing it had lost his only son, named Hamlet. As Sachs put it, 'Hamlet is what Shakespeare might have been if he had not written the play.'[2]

I was reminded, when Maxine told me about this reading of *Hamlet*, of my father and his love of Shakespeare – of his oft knee-jerk Shakespearean quoting. 'Two truths are told as prologues to the swelling act of the imperial theme!' he is wont to shout, upon the climax of a dinner-table story. 'Out, damned spot!' he will say in the kitchen as he tries to empty a bottle of tomato passata into a saucepan. Comical as those utterances are, it was the rich depth of metaphor in Shakespearean work that hooked him – there was for him no better symbol for unconscious guilt than Lady Macbeth's imagined blood-stained hands.

He had, while my mother was poring over *Hamlet*, begun his first year of university by correspondence, and had chosen, to befit his interest in the undiscovered self, psychology. Psychoanalysis must have been inextricably bound for him with a kind of European exoticism: I have a photo of my father in a trench coat in Leicester Square on a trip around the time he met my mother. Psychoanalysis would have linked him with a continental lifestyle of great appeal to a young man interested in a world beyond land-locked Johannesburg.

It also hinted at Aaron's burgeoning knowledge that there was a mystery at the heart of himself. But exposing that took a while yet, another decade – one in which Aaron and Maxine married and had Joni and then me, and then divorced.

3

They were renovating the hospital where I checked in for the settling program when Reuben was four months old. Beside the rooms where on the first night I would be granted the reprieve of uninterrupted sleep stood an earthmover. I glared at it hatefully as we entered the building, certain of its persecutory intention. Noise interruptions had become my nemesis. I cast fiery glances at road workers and muttered curses on people using leaf-blowers in our street.

Reuben's pattern, day or night, was to drift off into 45-minute snatches of quiet, before waking with a call that triggered a tension in me that did not cease until I put him on my breast. He was strong of voice as well as of body, and it was a howl that could not, as the nurses and midwives assured me, be considered a grizzle any more than an earthquake could be considered a rockfall. Another mother, a mother with less cortisol coursing through her veins, might have received the call with less alarm, might have picked him up and cuddled him and tucked him back in his cot, might have even had a drink of water or put her book away or eaten a bite of lunch. But the sound had a visceral effect on me; it terrified me – I felt if I didn't give him my breast immediately he would die from abandonment.

I had recorded the sound of his cry on my phone and I played it to our doctor, to the nurse we took him to for check-ups. Both suggested we might benefit from a settling program. In the 45-minute dips when he lapsed into rest I played it to myself, watching the decibel lines dart up jaggedly. I found it curious the way his recorded sound made my adrenalin leap even while he slept quietly beside me. Because his cry had this effect on me, I was constantly engaged in unsustainable acts to stave it off: I sat for hours in positions that cramped my arms and hands and strained my neck, lest I move when he was peaceful. I drove in circuits over the same bumpy roads, lest he wake from the car stopping. I breastfed and breastfed and breastfed, because when he was sucking he was content. It was not viable or helpful to either of us.

We had been on a waiting list for the settling program for a few weeks – short compared to other parents' wait, but seeming endless with my enduring panic. This sort of comparative assessment of my fortune had become a mental tic for me, useful in the same way that watching grotesque documentaries on morbid diseases might be to a person who fears death.

The wait had felt interminable. Every minute I longed to close my eyes and sleep, to get away from myself. When Reuben napped in the day, or slept in his hourly snatches at night, instead of drifting off myself I lay waiting for his cry, my pulse quickening. I feared the moment he needed me; that I wouldn't go.

Sometimes at night I went into his room and sat in the chair in the dark, awake, preferring to be right there when he called out than to be jolted from sleep, which felt to me like those nightmares I had where I was in a plane that started plummeting.

I couldn't engage my mind with anything much beyond surviving my own feelings. My imagined maternity leave – in which I would finally write regularly, read all the books I had sitting on my bedside table – had been usurped by a cruel regimen of clock-watching, mental tallying and googling, which I had put in place to quiet the panic. *White noise, sleep through, day routine,* I searched, convinced that if I could just get some decent sleep my mind would reset back to the old me. I kept a list of things that had triggered my crying, hoping to unlock a pattern: *When Brian*

Cox explained the Theory of Relativity. When opening a can of tomatoes. When the dog looked at me. When the stovetop coffeepot ring melted. When the doctor asked, What can I do for you? *When Gideon put his hand on my waist. When not a single pen worked.*

I wasn't sure if this trough I was in was normal new motherhood. I had no experience of looking after a baby, and very little exposure to new mothers. I'd barely held a baby before. Few of my friends had had babies yet and I had grown up without extended family around me. The antenatal classes we had attended had been highly theoretical – like learning to burp and change a rockmelon.

The how-to baby books had caused me alarm. Without a real baby to practise on I'd been unable to meaningfully absorb any of the information. The baby gurus had confounded me. Penelope Leach had read to me like a *Choose Your Own Adventure* through an Escher landscape, with headings like 'Sleeping and waking variations in the first three months', followed by subheading after subheading offering alternate options for settling a baby, followed by dot points and key questions and more options and smaller headings, all in a soft tone indicating that in any case all of this was entirely optional and questionable and not to be taken as advice. I knew that no book was going to impart the reality of the experience, and I had avoided imagining it too extensively.

I had wanted not manuals but narratives of motherhood, though I was no less determined that each narrative should tell me exactly what I wished to hear. Which is where I had gotten stuck. Rachel Cusk's memoir of early motherhood, *A Life's Work: on becoming a mother*, had frightened me. I had read many reviews of the book, the accusations that she did not love her children, that she was selfish – it wasn't those opinions that bothered me about it (I thought the reviewers lacked insight). It was that it confirmed my worst fears: that I might be entering a state of not-knowing, and that the task ahead of me was to find my way out. I had hidden that book away and become much more selective about the literature I chose. It needed to reflect my hopes. I googled: *books about motherhood being good; mothers who love being a mother*. I did not read Anne Enright's *Making Babies*, billed as being about 'the mess, the glory, and the raw shock of motherhood', or Adrienne Rich's *Of Woman Born*, whose introduction explains that, of new motherhood, Rich 'could remember little except anxiety, physical weariness, anger, self-blame, boredom, and division within myself'.

I'd moaned to my friends that no one had written a positive experience of motherhood. I'd complained to my mother that all the articles I read about parenthood only complained – about sleeplessness and unsettled babies and the demands of infants. *Why*, I asked her, *would anyone begrudge attending to their most beloved person, even at 2 am?* I'd loped around in this state of magical thinking – one in which a reality of difficulty or unpleasantness would be more than disappointing; it would topple me over the edge of my unacknowledged ambivalence.

I had been willing to read about the difficult task of childbirth itself, which would be over comparatively quickly. I'd happily sought out stories of precipitous labours on highways, munched on chips while reading about pelvic-floor tearing. Knowing other people's stories about childbirth excited me – I'd wanted very much to meet my baby, very much wanted a baby of my own. But, finding it impossible to imagine myself with one, I had focused, instead, on pregnancy, on my physiological state of growing another person, more than on the eventual arrival and care of that other person as a sentient being in the world beyond my womb. I had pushed away the vague, threatening sense that change – undefinable but enormous change – loomed. In pregnancy I had been on a train shuttling through a captivating wilderness without any sense that I would need at some point to alight and find a means to live in an alien land.

But in sleep, my mind had owned up to things: I'd had nightmare after nightmare about my dog drowning; in them, though, she was always a puppy – my child-self succumbing to the torrential pull of a body of water; it was both the baby waiting to be born in me and my adult self waiting to arrive. It did not occur to me until many years later, when I could see it all again behind me, that I was living the experience already; that the books were a mere distraction from witnessing myself already transformed.

So I had held at bay some grim truths about the difficulties of this parenting thing, but was that all this was? Me acclimatising to reality?

I doubted it. I had a history of reality turning irretrievably bad. I had been seeing a psychoanalyst, Dr Parkes, twice a week for five years, and I had begun to see him in the first place because a creeping ennui in me had similarly transformed. Everything had been going well in my life – I had met Gideon, for one, fallen in love. I adored Melbourne. I was gainfully employed, had friends. But I'd begun waking with free-floating dread, and one day it was not just when I woke but all the time. My stalling career as an underpaid journalist snowballed into an existential crisis, and into a variety of panic that seemed to mobilise my propensity to cry. On a trip to England with Gideon I had stood in phone boxes in Leicester Square and Covent Gardens and Camden while he went to work meetings, punching in my sister's phone number, then my mother's, then my father's, desperate to get hold of a voice that would tether me back to equilibrium so I could get out and enjoy the city. My father had given me the name of Dr Parkes.

In the years I had chipped away at the layers of my mind, lying on the analytic couch with Dr Parkes seated behind me, I had found out so much about myself, in that strange, broken talking that I did there: how I bowed to authority, how I feared my own rage. I had begun to learn to be myself there. I had felt, by the time I fell pregnant with Reuben, that I was rid of whatever it was that had caused me to turn good into bad.

Just before Reuben's birth, I had told Dr Parkes I wanted to take a four-week break from my appointments with him. 'I think it will be hard to be anywhere at a specific time,' I reasoned.

Though I was completely ignorant of the tasks involved in getting myself and a small baby out of the house, I could at least predict that making it across town for an 8 am appointment was unlikely after a broken night's sleep.

In that first week home, when I had suspected I was crying too much, I had phoned him. 'I am not too well,' I sobbed, with huge understatement.

'Do you feel you need to be in hospital?' he asked me.

I didn't know what going to hospital would do. I imagined gurneys and sedatives and my baby boy tinged green by fluorescent light. Instead, I'd rescheduled a weekly appointment, where I now went to sit in the russet velvet armchair opposite him instead of lying on the russet velvet chaise longue, holding Reuben or feeding Reuben, and staining Dr Parkes's antimacassars with tears and breast milk in equal measure. Lying down, facing away from the analyst, was a practice suggested by Freud to enable the patient to say what came to her, rather than feeling the need to respond to the cues of the analyst. It also prevented the patient from seeing the analyst's actual personage: if the analyst was a blank slate, a *tabula rasa*, the patient would much more easily come to project their own ingrained feelings and ways of relating onto them, as Freud suggested that we all do once those feelings have been embedded in our unconscious in early life. He called this *transference*. The main task of analysis is to identify this transference and bring it to light. Dr Parkes had never told me to lie on the couch, and in my first weeks of seeing him I had sat in the armchair. Then one day I had overcome my self-consciousness about the cliché of it all, and had lain on the couch instead.

I couldn't articulate anything much to Dr Parkes anyway on my return as a mother, in a chair or couch or hammock; I howled and cried and went through box after box of the tissues that sat on his desk, which I kept forgetting to bring myself and which began to provide a focus point for our discussions. 'I'm sorry; I need you to pass me some tissues,' I'd say, between sobs, my nose running. 'You don't feel you can get up and take them for yourself? You need to apologise?' he'd ask. A year later, when I was much better but then discovering my anger at him for the way I felt he had let me suffer during this time, I strode across the room forcefully and grabbed a handful of the tissues before returning in a huff to the armchair and blowing my nose with an aggressive honk.

There were days where I did talk, where I brought to him what was happening to me as best I could, but often what he suggested came from observing me. 'You cracked the knuckle on your left ring finger when you spoke,' he once noted as I talked about the night, how Reuben had cried out every thirty minutes, how I had spent most of it wide awake on his bedroom floor anticipating his next cry. 'The anxiety was worse if I got back into the bed with Gideon. I thought I was going to throw up. It was bearable if I stayed in Reuben's room,' I told him.

'Reuben is a third party to your marriage, as you see it.'

I gritted my teeth. 'What do you mean? I don't see what you are saying.' I often could not grasp his interpretations at first.

Silence. 'I'm not saying it; you are. You were twisting your wedding ring.'

'A baby is not a third party. I mean, it's not an affair,' I shot back indignantly. I was angry with him a lot, in between my crying.

'Just after you were born, your father found a third party,' he said. And when I thought about that I could see that the anxiety I felt away from Reuben had shadows of the anxiety I felt about my mother being alone after my father left. I was unable to let my baby know my absence, know my inability to meet his every need, my inability to be available to him at every moment. The famous analyst Donald Winnicott said of mother–baby relations that the mother, whom he calls 'the good-enough mother', one who is functioning well enough, 'starts off with an almost complete adaptation to her infant's needs, and as time proceeds she adapts less and less completely, gradually, according to the infant's growing ability to deal with her failure'.[3] I was projecting onto Reuben my own childhood fear: that Maxine's sadness would prevent her attending to me.

Silence. A session would go on like this until we threaded together an idea about my feelings.

I always felt better after a session. Calmer; I sometimes even laughed or felt hungry, eating a handful of the chocolate and nut biscuits a good baker friend of mine had delivered to me in old Danish biscuit tins.

Some days, too, I felt almost okay – when Reuben was a few weeks old we went to a wedding in the country. Aaron, visiting from Perth, came with us and stayed back at our motel with Reuben. The ceremony was at an art gallery, and the hard marble surfaces, the clinking glasses and caviar-heaped canapés were a stark contrast from the softness of baby skin and wool and blankets and pillows that my world had become. I experienced a jolting thrill of adulthood. I wolfed down the hors d'oeuvres, feeling I had regained some appetite, and was enlivened by the freezing night air when I drove back to the motel to feed Reuben.

The postbox panic had lost a bit of its steely sharpness; I'd forced myself to eat bowls of soup with meatballs in them, which Joni had stocked our freezer with in the week she flew out from Sydney, where she lived with her husband, to meet her new nephew and witness her crumbling sister. I was still reeling with the hurt of my mother absconding back to Sydney. My mother, my mother, my mother. Never before had I needed my mother so badly and she had flown back 900 kilometres from me because she was angry with my father. Was she punishing me for becoming a mother, for leaving her in the biggest way a daughter can? Or had watching me as a mother brought back such untenably painful memories for her that she could not bear it? Joni's presence was an anchor; she sat with me for hours at a time while I cried, reminding me over and over again that nothing was going to happen to me beyond feelings. She was two years older than me, and though she hadn't had a baby herself she was a nurse, well-versed in matters of the body. I was experiencing the effects of adrenalin, cortisol. I was not, in fact, being swallowed by a sinkhole.

I had hoisted a safety net of obsessive record-keeping to stop myself from falling: every time I fed Reuben, I wrote down which breast he had started on, and the time. I followed the instructions of my home-visiting nurse to a tee, ensuring I put him on both breasts. He was full as a piglet, gaining 300 grams a week. The visiting nurse clucked at this, sighed, 'Wow, Nicola. Wo-o-w.' She had seen me during the postbox panic; her determination to assure me of my competency as a mother was touching. I also wrote down the time he drifted off to sleep and the time he woke. The list began to fill a spiral notebook. It reminded me of the list I had kept as a teenager, turning to food restriction to stave off the unpredictable awfulness that was the domestic warfare of my mother's second marriage: *1 yoghurt – 0.5 g fat; 1 apple – 0 grams fat.*

In between my record-keeping of Reuben's feeding and sleep, I tallied up my own sleep. It felt essential to my not succumbing to the panic that I get at least six hours in a 24-hour cycle. I kept a ledger of these broken hours in the notebook. I got into bed the moment Gideon came home from work, to rack up at least one hour. I handed Reuben to him, climbed under the covers and finally felt my shoulders drop, the release of an hour or so in which I knew the baby was the safest he could be, lying on my husband's chest, in the dark of the lounge listening to classical music. I had no idea if Gideon ate dinner; I had dropped all pretence of mutual care. This was survival.

Later, once we had bathed Reuben and I had fed him and wrapped him and laid him in his cot, I returned to bed, where I forced the dog into a kind of body-lock, and covered our heads with the doona to mute the world. I could not read. Before I was a mother I had read countless manuscripts every day in my work and then returned home to read books for pleasure. But now I could not take in a single word on paper. Even on my phone, I could not follow long sentences. A curtain had dropped on my seeing. Fiction, particularly, caused my faculties to shut down. Once I had written short stories but now I felt rage toward fiction writers for their gratuitous task. Life felt urgent; there was no time for art.

Nor could I listen to the hundreds of messages friends had left on my phone. Like the presents piling up on the dining table, they were a reminder of all I was supposed to be feeling: celebratory, in communion. Instead, I would close my eyes, recount the hours I had slept that day, and plunge wholly into a dark sanctuary. Often, just before I fell asleep I hallucinated that I could see into Reuben's room, that he was able to sit up, that he was looking for me.

I was comforted by how in love I felt with Reuben – even with the inexplicable lurching dread that washed over me when I opened my eyes each morning, there was a glint of excitement to feel knowing that he was mine forever. But there was resentment too, for the unrelenting attendance I made to him; a worry that the calm I felt when he finally drifted off to sleep was a sign that I wished he wasn't there. I confessed this to my father over the phone one night. 'His Majesty the Baby,' he said, reminding me of the phrase Freud had used in talking about the necessary narcissism of babies, who depend upon their parents to attend to their needs in early life as a matter of survival. 'Talking about your ambivalence is important,' he said, reminding me of Winnicott's theory that acknowledged maternal ambivalence helps babies with their own emotional development, their own ability to tolerate bad feelings. Ambivalence in psychoanalytic terms wasn't a lack of caring either way; it was deep hatred and deep love coexisting. One couldn't exist without the other, according to Freud.

I feared that Reuben wasn't sleeping because of something that I was doing to him or not doing to him. And of course I was acutely aware, but in a distant, disbelieving way, that his sleep patterns might be in cahoots with my permanent state of panic. That perhaps encountering a mother who looms over your bassinet with fear in her eyes when you voice a mere burp is not conducive to drifting back off to sleep peacefully.

During the day, once the initial cold adrenalin of morning had passed, I felt close to happy holding Reuben in the new spring sunlight. He slept in the crook of my arm while I watched a TV show about a comically dreamy obstetrician. I found, though, even when I watched TV, my thoughts were moored to my predicament. Did the actress playing the obstetrician have children? Did their cries cause her to break into a cold sweat? Was it true to life that the characters going home with their new babies were smiling and not crying?

The panic was much less pronounced when Reuben was with me; it was at night when he was separate from me that I felt it, when the prospect of the next day loomed like a tidal wave.

Back in this more recent trough I was coping better, in that I was now used to my permanent state of panic and not in a panic about the panic itself, but Reuben would still not sleep for any long stretch. It was with this superficial point that I tricked myself into attending the hospital's residential settling program. *Oh, no,* I assured family and friends, *we're going to Sleep School; I'm fine.* I struggled to recognise that my mental state was not going to be fixed by a magic wand of perfect routine; it seemed to me if I could get Reuben to sleep regularly and predictably, I would go back to feeling like my old self.

Sleep School was, as the brochures put it, where parents went when their babies hadn't learned how to resettle themselves after they rose into a light sleep during their REM cycle. It was where parents of chronically colicky babies went, even though through my incessant googling I knew well that colic was not a thing that could be cured but merely a word for a baby who will not settle. Sleep School was for parents like me to unlearn the *bad habits* they had gotten into that were inextricably linked to their deprived mental faculties. Sleep School had been named thus to assure parents like me, who were on a knife's edge, that there was something practical they could learn that would improve things. It suited my continued bid to convince myself that my mental state was nothing more than the result of exhaustion.

Gideon seemed relieved that we were going. He was by nature defiantly patient and optimistic and rarely acknowledged grave depths of feeling in himself. He was the sort of person who would be swept away by a tornado still smiling and assuring me that it was only a strong wind. He had taken on the British reserve that ran through his family, keeping sadness and anxiety under tight rein. Any pedestrian stress or boredom he felt was resolved by baking a cake or watching sport or reading about sport.

Given how different we were in this respect, he had been amazingly supportive of my newly unhinged self, always taking my sobbing midday phone calls at his open-plan workplace with gentility. Never once had he hung up on me. Which is not to say we did not fight. The combined stresses of my fragile self, sleep deprivation, and our opposing sense of how to handle Reuben's wakefulness gave way to heated arguments. I seemed to have developed the sonar hearing of a bat, and I demanded to know why Gideon never seemed to wake to Reuben crying at night, why it always had to be me to go to him; but I also criticised whatever he did in his efforts to settle Reuben when he did go. 'You're jostling him too much; it's actually waking him!' 'Stop making that *sh* sound in his ear – it's too loud!'

I couldn't understand why he couldn't understand how terrified I felt when Reuben would not stop crying, and he couldn't understand why I couldn't let Reuben cry a bit. I begged for his help in settling Reuben at night, but then when Reuben did not settle with him immediately (used, as Reuben was, to my breast appearing in his mouth at the slightest *peep*), I would rush in and wrestle Reuben from him and breastfeed Reuben and cry and then blame Gideon for his failed attempt. Once, at the peak of this insane parental warfare, I threw a toasted panini at Gideon's head.

In the text messages he sent me, even in their brevity – *Okay? Love you* – I saw that Gideon was scared for me, for us, but I also saw that he was angry with me. I was now back to twice-weekly analysis appointments with Dr Parkes: 'Why isn't it helping you?' he would ask. I felt ashamed of how much of an expense it was for us, too, and worried that Gideon would resent that. Though I had negotiated a fee I could afford, it was still a chunk of our earnings.

Gideon's understanding of psychoanalysis was limited to the time I had insisted we watch a Woody Allen movie. It had become a joke between us that he would ask, when I returned from seeing Dr Parkes, 'So...what did you talk about?' and I would roll my eyes and that would be the end of the conversation.

It was almost impossible to describe to someone else what went on in analysis. It was piecemeal; it was so often banal, fragmentary. The novelist Marie Cardinal had written that it would 'take thousands of pages, many of them repetitious, in order to express the interminability of nothingness, the emptiness, the vagueness, the slowness, the deadness, the essential and the perfectly simple'.[4] Winnicott had put it this way, from the analyst's perspective: 'It is difficult to report analytical material. First, there is the immensity of the task of remembering an hour's work and then of writing it down. Second, there is the quantity of material and the difficulty there must be in choosing from it. Third, there is the special difficulty analysts seem to find in recording what they themselves said.'[5]

Freud in the first place had struggled with how to convey the analytic process to someone who had not been in analysis, saying that it was 'to be regretted that we cannot let them be present as an audience at a treatment of this kind'.[6]

Sometimes, before Reuben was born, before I had stopped being able to read, I'd find a description of analysis and highlight it, tear it out, read it out loud to Gideon.

'Listen!' I'd say.

I read him what the analyst Neville Symington said: 'I can tell you about Freud, who was the first psychoanalyst and who gave us its name. I can tell you about the topographic model of the mind, the concepts of resistance, repression or transference … but you will not be an inch nearer knowing what psychoanalysis *is*. Psychoanalysis is a phenomenon which occurs at the centre of the individual. So when I say you cannot be taught psychoanalysis it is because it can occur only through a personal act of understanding.'[7]

I read him a scene from Patrick White's *Riders in the Chariot*, which was not about psychoanalysis at all but in which I'd found in the interaction between the damaged loner Miss Hare and the Holocaust survivor Himmelfarb something that felt like the analytic relationship. Miss Hare, who has suffered traumas and lacks a language to know herself, begins to see that it is this not-knowing that damns her: 'Eventually I shall discover what is at the centre, if enough of me is peeled away,' she says.[8] Later she recognises in Himmelfarb a listener who might help her understand herself, who will not resist meaning on account of pain, even though Himmelfarb himself isn't sure of this. She is willing to sit with him through his painful story too. '"I know," she said, gently for her, "I know that, probably, the worst bits are to come. But I shall endure them with you. Two," she said, "are stronger than one."'[9]

'Uh-huh,' Gideon had offered.

'Oh, wait! Here!' I yelled into the bathroom one evening as Gideon showered. 'It's from the book I'm reading; Vivian Gornick: "I walked into an analyst's office. I told her everything. I told her everything again. And then again. Whenever I told her everything she said: Why?"'[10]

He came out the bathroom, drying himself. 'So you pay to be asked a lot of questions?'

Though I could not explain to Gideon how, seeing Dr Parkes had changed me. More than I could ever have imagined.

Ψ

Now, settled in my bleak room beside the earthmover, Reuben and I were assessed by doctors, paediatricians and a psychologist. The latter gave me a piece of paper with a questionnaire: the Edinburgh Postnatal Depression Scale. Ten multiple-choice questions that in tone reminded me of the Monty Python 'Dead Parrot' sketch, so avoidant was their tentative expression of my clear inner doom: 'I have been able to laugh and see the funny side of things *not quite so much now*; I have looked forward with enjoyment to things *rather less than I used to*; I have felt scared or panicky for no very good reason *quite a lot*; I have been so unhappy that I have been crying *quite often*.'

The psychologist tallied my score and considered me gravely. 'You know,' she said, 'we can admit you. Just get you on an even keel; eating, sleeping.'

Some vague part of me had known all along that the program also catered to maternal mental health, but I had continued to deny it to myself, still unable to acknowledge that among the two kinds of mothers there, the hollowed-out, shocked-looking ones and the simply tired-looking ones, I was among the former. Out in the communal area, one woman seemed to float beside a nurse, looking but not seeing while the nurse tried to calm her baby. That baby never stopped its wretched cry in the three days we were there; I got used to its sound as I did to the constant low air-conditioning hum. But I failed to see myself in that mother, because Reuben was nothing like that baby. He was calm, and settled, and I would hold him all day if it killed me.

We stayed for our three nights, with Gideon visiting each evening. I told him what I had learned each day about Reuben's needs, how he seemed to sleep well when the nurses rolled him on his side, how they had suggested I increase his food intake. I told him about the feeding schedule the nurses had drawn up for us, and showed him the patting and shushing technique we were to use when it wasn't a feeding-time wake-up. I later learned this technique was the holy measure of parental competency for those who aligned themselves neither with co-sleeping nor with crying it out. Gideon listened patiently, employed the technique effortlessly. But it still felt as though the baby and I were in some netherworld which Gideon could visit but not enter.

At night, I was supposed to rely on the nurses to bring Reuben to me when they couldn't settle him. But it was this very separation, this severing of the soundwaves connecting me to my child that I couldn't tolerate. I asked to have a monitor in my room, and they acquiesced, the nurse who plugged it in looking at me with what might have been pity or, I later thought, resignation; I was not one who would be easily helped.

During the days, I sat with the other shipwrecked mothers in a waiting area of couches positioned facing a cluster of numbered audio monitors. Despite our exhaustion, we attended those monitors with uncanny alertness. It was heliotropic, all those maternal heads turning toward the bellows from those machines, and if the cry was our child's and it was not a scheduled feeding time, we received nods of support and encouragement that carried us over to our baby's room where we put to work our new strategy. I was a diligent student and, probably sensing his mother had found a rope to cling to, Reuben did indeed settle quite contentedly without my breast.

But I could not give myself over to hospital care as the psychologist had offered. I felt I was not sick enough: I had a comparative glut of therapeutic help. I felt almost ashamed taking the space in this hospital, with these mothers who seemed to be being taught how to love their babies, when I loved my baby achingly, overwhelmingly. And when I had my very own analyst at hand with his tear-dampened chaise longue. I felt I would embarrass my family and Gideon's family and disappoint Gideon, who had been trying so hard to carry on with life as though his wife hadn't suffered a malfunction, bringing takeaway Thai and magazines to the hospital like we were on some kind of getaway. I felt that close at hand but hidden from me was the source of my panic: if I could just find it, with the help of Dr Parkes, and bring it to light safely, I would be okay; I was sure.

I took the sleeping pill they offered me each night in the confines of my quasi-hotel room, where the oak veneers and complimentary biscuits abetted my delusion that I was not in hospital, and glided off into the glassy surface of its kind of sleep, which I rose from only briefly each time Reuben cried out.

4

Once, when I was in kindergarten, a girl came and stood beside me as I launched myself up and down on the seesaw. She said to me, 'Your father loves me more than he loves you.' I hadn't expected the spokesperson for my hidden fears to materialise in a playground. Nor had I yet recognised those hidden fears. That came later, when I wondered, as an adult, why Aaron and I always signed our letters to each other with the made-up initialism *N.E.K.*, which stood for *Never-Ending Kisses*: was it that we were both aware of an alternate turn of events for us in which they could have ended? Or why as a child I had carted around a shrunken tracksuit top Aaron had worn in 1985, with a diagonal zip and a fluorescent stripe, surreptitiously sniffing it when I felt sad.

The girl, it turned out, was a patient of my father's. Aside from whether her words held any truth – which my father assured me, in the car on the way home from school that day, they did not – the fact remained that she had allotted swathes of time alone in Aaron's company.

Later, in Australia, as a teenager, I would gain a more nuanced sense of the significance of the time these mystery people spent with my father. Once, visiting Aaron for the holidays, we went for the morning to some markets. We were browsing a book stall when a woman came up to greet him. He behaved strangely to her, I thought; he was aloof, controlled, and he did not introduce me. He guided me away to a different stall.

'She's a patient of mine,' he eventually said. This happened again from time to time – at a party, the pool. I felt from these exchanges there was a rule about how he could relate to his patients, a pact of privacy, or a decree on friendship between them. But for all his aloofness to them, I saw signs from his patients of deep attachment to him, even love. Patients had made him extraordinary artworks: delicate paper cuttings and sculptures. At Christmas time they baked him biscuits, bottled jams. Sometimes the phone would ring and my father would have to go to another room to talk, and when he returned he would explain that it had been a patient. These people needed my father.

Before all that, still back in Johannesburg, his work had become compelling to me, possibly from simple envy at a growing realisation that my father spent his days attending to the emotions of other people – and in those days, many children, since my father then specialised in child psychotherapy. Who came to see him in his *rooms*, as he called the cottage behind his house, with its particular smell that would later move with him from Johannesburg to Perth and then Melbourne; the smell I associated with new paint, wool, pen ink and a hint of his woody aftershave. And what did he do with those people who came to see him?

The cottage, with its opaque net curtains and heavy sliding doors, shut me outside its borders during the week, when I watched it through a chink in the curtains if Joni and I went there after school. But on the weekends that my sister and I stayed with him I investigated warily the interior, where I was allowed to play freely in the sandpit, use the stick-on farm scenes or even paint if I wished. The room had been set up for him to observe children at play, and I thought the space strangely lonely, the sense of another child's quiet time with my father sorrowful. Later I recognised that my feelings for those children was misplaced: it was sorrow for my own loss of time with him that I could not bear to own.

I found the remnants of those troubled children's play – the half-formed sandcastles and dried up Play-Doh – abject, almost icky. They held the trace of a stranger's intimacy. I sensed that, in the room with my father, part of his work was to let the strangers be wild; to spill their tears or sickness or anger. The world of my father's work – dreams and the observed play of children and the indents left in chairs by sad grown-ups – seemed to be filled with experiences that were both compelling and spooky for me: it was like coming upon dead things that spoke, or finding that a seemingly meaningless cluster of letters was a code for a treasure map. Uncanny, is the word Freud might have used for it: that which unconsciously reminds us of our own locked-away impulses.

I already had a compulsion for unveiling hidden messages. Joni and I spent countless hours each day playing detectives in our house in central Johannesburg, a short drive from Aaron's house. The brutal Apartheid system was expected to end; there was a fear of revolution. Anti-Apartheid activists were being disappeared into prison; bastions of white nationalism were being bombed by the African National Congress, the underground anti-Apartheid movement whose president, Nelson Mandela, lingered in prison on Robben Island. I knew little of this intellectually, but something of the fear around me had permeated my child world. There was the story of a white girl who had held up her hand in the fist sign of the ANC in the back of her parents' car, and had been arrested; there were the bomb threats at school.

Perhaps we had absorbed the country's paranoia: we looked at the old telephone tower that loomed over our suburb through binoculars, turning any object into a vital clue to our invented criminal activity. Wet jeans flapping in the wind on a balcony were bloodstained, a dark object on the balcony rail a gun.

That spark of omniscience, the feeling of being the one to gather together the disparate evidence, infiltrated the rest of my life. I longed to engage my father in an un-riddling of his mind, to find out what no one spoke about openly: what had happened to cause him to not live with my mother and my sister and me? Psychoanalytic thinking, in the limited way I understood it as a child, was a wormhole into understanding my own often inexplicable loss and fear and even joy.

Not long after that little girl came up to me, the night before my sixth birthday party, Aaron's father, Perry, died. He had a heart attack in the hotel suite he lived in with my grandmother, Bella, where you could go to the restaurant any time of day and get kipper and eggs or borscht or jelly and ice cream. The hotel loomed above Johannesburg city, filled with elderly people suffering coronaries in its quiet, muffled rooms. It was endlessly interesting to me, with fake Renaissance art in the lounge where the residents played competitive Bridge – including a copy of Bruegel's *The Peasant Wedding* scene with its confounding extra foot – and a man named Pumpkin who operated the lift and explained to me that the building had no floor thirteen, out of superstition.

Joni and I happened to be spending that weekend at Aaron's house, and the next morning I woke up in his bed, where I had gone in the middle of the night after waking, scared. My father was crying. I had never seen him cry before. He told me my grandmother had called an ambulance but they couldn't get my grandfather's heart working again. His voice sounded different, squeezed.

It was alarming to see my father cry, to bear the knowledge that fathers died and fathers trailed snot out their noses and fathers shook with grief.

Someone covered the mirrors of the art-deco house Aaron shared with his flatmate Paul, and my father stopped shaving. Perry was buried within a day, according to Jewish tradition. They cancelled my party, although one boy turned up because no one had been able to get hold of his parents, and I felt disproportionate shame about letting him down. It was one way of filtering my own untenable sadness.

My father's siblings flew in from the UK the next morning. Our family had already begun to scatter around the globe in early anticipation of a violent end to white rule. Later his lounge room filled with people, and the rabbi arrived, and my father swayed alongside his brother and said *Kaddish* for their father, and people lined up to wish my grandfather's wife and children 'long life'. Family and friends brought an inordinate amount of food in accordance with the customs of *shiva*, the seven days of mourning. They brought cakes, sandwiches, breads, stews and biscuits; it all fanned out across Aaron's Indian teak dining-room table. I was not at the prayers, being too young, but the fathers and sons I've seen since, pale and unshaven, their clothes rent, often stumbling over the *Kaddish*, Hebrew words they had hoped never to say, have moved into my memory as though I was.

I got a World Book encyclopaedia set that same year, which I kept at Maxine's house. I was drawn to the entry on the human body in volume H, especially to the heart. Unlike the other plain pages of glossy paper, this entry had a special insert – three films of see-through paper that revealed in layers the venal system, the bones and the organs.

There was a see-through page soon overlaid onto my memories of waking in the bed next to my father crying, too. Three years after my grandfather's death, when I was nine years old, in an elevator with Aaron and Joni, heading down to somewhere that I have blanked out, but let's say a shopping centre (or perhaps it wasn't in a lift at all but rather what he said that caused a sensation of plummeting), my father told me something about himself that changed how I understood my place in that bed beside him that morning. It was not my place: it was Paul's. And when Joni and I weren't there on the weekends, it was his and Paul's room. He said, and he was crying again: 'I am gay.'

There are a few versions of how I remember responding to my father's news that day. In one, I am curiously unaffected, having already worked through the shock of this revelation the day I discovered a Hallmark card saying *I Love You* next to his bed and signed by his purported flatmate Paul, whose purported bedroom was that with the light blue linen and white lace down the hall from my father's. In another, I am again upset at seeing my father cry, and prioritise assuring him of my okay-ness, while later that night in my own bedroom burning hot with an anxiety that what my father had told me about himself was a secret I must maintain with great effort.

It was 1987 and my sister and mother and I had emigrated to Australia two years before. Now my father had finally emigrated too, and Paul. Paul felt like family and treated Joni and me as his children – he plaited my long hair and painted my face like a cat for a dress-up party. Aaron must have known it was no longer plausible to maintain the idea of such a dedicated flatmate. Also, Joni and I were growing up: soon enough we would realise the implications of all those weekends we'd spent with them listening to Queen and watching videos of Baryshnikov dancing, all the tennis-playing my father and Paul did with other well-maintained and moustachioed male twosomes. The lace in Paul's bedroom, his floral arrangements and manicured hands.

In our new home in Australia, the government had started screening ads on television depicting the grim reaper bowling down men, women, children. 'At first only gays and IV drug users were being killed by AIDS. But now we know every one of us could be devastated by it,' the ad ran. Being openly gay and a dad at the same time was a rarity then. Gayness presupposed a vastly disparate lifestyle from that of the Jewish family man my father had been until he came out. Gayness was flamboyant: Boy George in his kaftans and Freddie Mercury with his tight white pants. It was not possible to be gay and picking up your kids from the sports carnival in an old Volvo. Later, as an adult, I learned that, back in South Africa, before I was aware of his sexuality, his coming out had been shocking in the staidly traditional Jewish community he and my mother had moved in. Couples composed largely of young Jewish men and women with parents who had come from Britain or Eastern Europe either as migrants or refugees during World War Two, and who were still feeling the after-effects of what had been a relatively recent obliteration of their forebears for being part of a group that was distinctly other. In Jewish South Africa, homosexuality was not quite taboo, but it was for homosexuals, as Maxine put it. 'We all knew gay men,' my mother explained to me now when I asked her. 'My hairdresser was effeminate, outright gay. But we all kept it quiet: if you were in the community gayness was concealed; gay men were considered confirmed bachelors. It was a whole different thing for a family man, a father in a marriage, to come out.'

Beyond their particular community, in the wider South African community, homosexuality was not talked about or expressed freely. The Dutch Reformed Church, the official religion of the white National Party during the Apartheid era, had shaped the cultural milieu, and it was a heavily Calvinistic kind of influence, marked by an idea of God as a deterministic force overseeing who was saved and who went to hell. As long as you adhered to the Church's teachings, you would be saved. South Africa's Apartheid-era treatment of gay people within the defence forces stands as an example of just how taboo it was in the institutional sphere. Gay men and women were subjected to untold abuses both through damaging psychological treatments such as exposure therapies using electric shocks and, horrifically, through forced gender reassignment surgery under the simplistic belief that this would therefore 'correct' their sexual preference.[11] When Paul had served in the army – still in his late twenties, having chosen to serve three weeks of every year as a commando, rather than the year of training Aaron had opted for as a seventeen-year-old – he and Aaron had written to each other using a female pseudonym for Aaron, to protect themselves.

The embarrassment and surprise I felt in hearing my father's confession that day in the elevator, whichever version I remember, did not come because I thought any less of him or Paul as a result of what I now knew concretely. They came because it was deemed necessary in the first place for him to treat the news as a revelation or secret, and because I, at the age of nine, was uncomfortable with the predicament of having my father relay information to me about his love life, full stop. Of same-sex attraction itself, I had little imagination to shock myself with. Maxine says now that she never had to explain to Joni and me how babies were made – we seemed to know. But I think we did not know. Sex, as far as I could conceive of it at that point, was only what I knew was *adults only* in Maxine's favourite shows: the heated mushing up of Michael Douglas's and Kathleen Turner's bodies in a wet jungle in *Romancing the Stone*; Bruce Willis and Cybill Shepherd locked in an embrace in *Moonlighting*. And I did not want to have any adult talk to me about it. But in the climate of the AIDS campaign, faced with an absence of gay representation in anything around me – there were no TV shows or books I saw where two men were partners – and Aaron's own clear distress at having to tell me this about himself, I decided that the news should be kept hidden; that the typically suburban clusters of ordinary parents that my friends had might recoil from our family if they knew, and I fretted about what my school mates might think. It was into that conventional version of shame that I projected all my intense feelings about what my father being gay meant about me. Later, as an adult, I found out that everyone who knew us knew anyway, and hardly anyone cared.

By the time he and Paul settled in Perth, my mother had remarried and we were relocating to Sydney. This meant I had to worry far less about hiding my father from my school friends. It was only a part-time worry: when we went back to Perth during school holidays. Then, I spent my time alone or with my sister or with children whom I met through my father's and Paul's adult friendships. A girl whose father had also come out after spending years in a monastery. A boy whose eccentric, itinerant parents built each new house by hand and only had gay friends. If I made friends outside of that world, I concocted elaborate excuses for why they could not come to play at my father's house. 'His house is so small,' I'd say. My father and Paul tacitly understood this arrangement: they never appeared together in front of these friends, and my father never mentioned Paul to my friends' parents when he collected me.

Decades later, when Reuben was born, when I held the irrefutable proof of how babies were made, I saw that my father being gay and contributing to my conception during a heterosexual marriage gave rise to complex existential questions about myself; that the not-feeling I had experienced in that elevator masked overwhelming doubt I had tucked away inside myself. How had my mother and father conceived me if my father wasn't attracted to women? Or was he sometimes attracted to women? Had he wanted another child? Was I a result of double deception, both my mother and father in full knowledge that the marriage would end? Or was I a last-ditch attempt at marital repair? I asked my mother one day. 'I knew something was very wrong,' she said. 'I thought it was that your father was depressed. He was cut off; absent. But we both adored being parents. We decided to have another baby. We both wanted another child. We tried for you once and I fell pregnant.' So, I was wanted. Whatever else was going on, they wanted to be parents. That was a relief.

What had my father known about himself? I had constructed an idealised version of my early life that I relayed to anyone enquiring of my family story: 'My parents divorced when I was a baby, but my father was incredibly present in our lives,' I would explain. 'He saw us every night for a bedtime story and every morning to take us to school,' I would say. I told this story as though the intervening night-time, the time when he should have been in bed beside my mother, was irrelevant to a marriage, to a family.

Now, in every small moment I saw Gideon with Reuben, the

early mornings when they lay stomach to stomach, the midnights when Gideon came to change Reuben's nappy after a feed while I went back to bed, I mourned my father's absence from my babyhood.

What did Aaron say to Maxine when he left? When I was twenty-six, the same age she was when he left, I fractured my hand on the way to the bathroom to shower. I turned the corner at an odd angle and my closed fist, clutching the clothes I had been wearing, slammed into the door frame at speed. I had an operation to put a metal plate in along the line where the bone cracked. Since then, a nervy shock runs along the resulting scar like electricity if I feel a very particular kind of emotion. If I am misunderstood or left out; if I hear about loss. I tried to explain it to Dr Parkes once – 'It's the sorrow of fathers leaving' was all I could come up with.

5

From Sleep School I got a new structure to cling to, and for the first week back home I had renewed vigour. The patting and shushing technique I had learned offered me a practical alternative to breastfeeding. I loved breastfeeding Reuben, the feeling of his body tucked into mine, the gentle sucking sound he made. But with Dr Parkes I had begun to see that constantly breastfeeding Reuben, while it might be perfectly suited to another mother–baby relationship, reinforced an unhelpful sense in me that he and I were one. Plus, I had realised while at Sleep School, I needed some other settling strategies for him on account of my physical exhaustion.

Although I had built up, while hunched over a machine that whirred and sucked uncomfortably from my nipples, a storehouse of tiny packets of frozen breastmilk in varying shades from bluish-white (*That's the foremilk, full of water*, the midwife had told me) to creamy yellow (*That's the hindmilk, full of fat*), Reuben would not take a bottle, eliminating Gideon from the feeding equation. Now Gideon could take more of a role at least in settling him, and in his quiet way he learned and enacted it perfectly. I watched him pat-pat-patting Reuben's blanketed shape and I saw, in his confident employment of this new technique, how hard it had probably been for him to fit into our knotted companionship; how I had barely left space between us for another parent. Perhaps, when he came home from work in his neat suit and pressed shirt, smelling of the outside world of trains and lunchtime rain and printer-ink, he felt painfully outside the borders of the baby's and my milk-sodden existence.

So Sleep School eased our resentments toward each other as parents, but its teachings only proved helpful to my anxiety on the days when they worked. Then, I felt I had some control. The problem was, they didn't always work. Often, no matter how long I stood over Reuben, my body bent unnaturally over the cot rail, my hands working their rhythm, he squirmed and fought and looked at me wide-eyed with near mirth. On those days, I felt even more helpless. On those days, I wondered if he was happier awake and I should let him be. But I was so tired myself that I longed for him to sleep so that I could. The nurses had sent me home with clear schedules for feeding, sleeping and playing time. *Feed, Play, Sleep.* In that mantra, my sleep-addled brain saw not commonsense that I could use flexibly, but a magical incantation that ought to be followed precisely. If I couldn't get him to settle again after forty-five minutes, if I failed at the patting and shushing, if we couldn't stick to the schedule, then I was lost again.

When the Sleep School technique failed, determined to stave off my feelings of helplessness, I performed feats of physical mastery. One wet end-of-summer day Gideon came home from work to find me walking the pram endlessly around the tiny deck outside our house, clothes soaked, pouring a can of baked beans into my mouth, my stomach empty from forgetting to eat all day. I often forgot to eat because I felt no hunger. Reuben was fast asleep, but I couldn't stop walking in case he woke before the schedule dictated.

I carried on daily in a strange position of both knowing and not knowing that I was functioning problematically. Partly this was because on paper I was highly competent. Reuben was growing fat; I loved him with tremendous sureness and felt certain of the bond we were developing. I adored his face, his body; I photographed him and examined the photographs endlessly when he did sleep, hardly believing I had given life to such a darling thing. I also felt able to verbalise and know my resentment of him, and was confident that this was a healthy way, a better way, to be than to be harbouring feelings of anger toward him. Winnicott's famous statement, which he had made about the role of the analyst in therapy as well as the mother, had stayed with me: 'However much he loves his patients he cannot avoid hating them and fearing them, and the better he knows this the less will hate and fear be the motives determining what he does to his patients.'[12]

My knowledge of psychoanalytic ideas delivered its own source of anxiety. The mother, according to British psychoanalyst Wilfred Bion, attends to her baby in a state he called 'reverie' – a state of receptive attunement – and responds with gestures that meet the baby's: he gurgles, she gurgles. Bion said this delivers the baby's feelings back to the baby in a digestible form and the baby feels comforted and satisfied. If she fails to attain a state of reverie – perhaps her own feelings of envy, depression or hatred toward the baby are so strong – she does not 'contain' the baby's projections. Instead, the baby experiences a sense of his being too much for her and internalises a bad sense of himself.[13]

I was hyper-aware of unwittingly conveying my distress to Reuben, of a need to keep myself in check. 'The baby quickly learns to make a forecast: *Just now it is safe to forget the mother's mood and to be spontaneous, but any minute the mother's face will become fixed or her mood will dominate, and my own personal needs must then be withdrawn otherwise my central self may suffer insult.* Immediately beyond this in the direction of pathology is predictability, which is precarious, and which strains the baby to the limits of his or her capacity to allow for events.'[14] I was constantly trying to deconstruct what my innermost unconscious feelings might be, what might be lurking beyond my awareness, so that I could respond to my baby's actual needs and not have them obscured by whatever I might be projecting onto him. This, in itself, was both exhausting and impossible, and served as its own kind of defence, putting me at a great distance from my actual feelings.

It is a paradox, after all, to think that I can know what I don't know about how I feel, but attempting it kept my mind distracted.

And there was Melanie Klein haunting me. Klein, who put forward a theory that the infant experiences their caregivers as part-objects: the mother's hand, the mother's breast and so on. Each object is experienced as split off from other objects, to allow the baby to tolerate their bad feelings when the whole object does not fulfill their needs. The bad breast can be tolerated if the rest of the mother is good. Healthy development, Klein suggested, must see the baby develop a strong enough sense of the reality of their caregiver as a whole, including the good and the bad. She called this the *depressive position*. What if I failed to allow Reuben to develop psychically because of my own emotional incapacities?

I had psychoanalytic theory rattling around in my head as a matter of course. I had grown up with it. Aaron was a psychotherapist who drew on psychoanalytic theory – what is known as a psychodynamic therapist. Maxine had moved away from her adolescent psychoanalytic interest and gone into health sciences, but her *lingua franca* had remained distinctly Freudian.

The names of the great analytic thinkers – Freud, Klein, Bowlby, Bion – had lined both my parents' bookshelves. My adolescent reading had been far from the romances my friends were absorbing at night under the covers; while they were secreting Virginia Andrews's tales of family incest I was reading those fictitious relations in Freud's theories of the Oedipus complex. I had devoured books on mental illness and recovery – *I Never Promised You a Rose Garden*, a semi-autobiographical novel about a girl named Deborah Blau who retreats to a fantasy world in which she is ruled by persecutory gods, and her recovery through psychoanalytic therapy; *Sybil*, about the psychoanalytic treatment of the pseudonymous Sybil, a woman with what was then called multiple personality disorder (dissociative identity disorder); *Dibs in Search of Self*, which chronicles the therapy of a severely emotionally impoverished little boy. Minds bid hidden treasures, concealed unconscious thought that would reveal itself in mysterious ways.

I drew what I could from my father about the work of the mind. On steaming days, while other children were running through Perth's sulfurous sprinkler water, I was getting my father to tell me about object-relations theory, or dream interpretation. Before that, as young as seven, I'd come to absorb something of the psychoanalytic process: Aaron had become a minor celebrity in Johannesburg, appearing on a weekly commercial radio show offering his psychoanalytic ear to callers. From my position at his feet in the dark under the switchboard desk of the radio station, I listened as people from all around the city phoned to seek help according to the topic of the week – dreams, childhood trauma, infidelity. I understood little of these callers' problems, but I took the essence of psychoanalysis from the conversations by osmosis. The talking, the listening, the stringing together of meaning. The sense that speaking and then understanding gave relief.

One summer, in a warm patch of sunlight on the old Persian rug in Aaron's consulting rooms, I read *The Words to Say It* by Marie Cardinal. In it, the narrator experiences continuous menstruation along with debilitating anxiety that she calls *the Thing*. 'The Thing that had rooted in my mind, this filthy hag whose two enormous buttocks were the lobes of my brain.' She begins psychoanalysis. The Thing, and her bleeding, is what she comes to understand as a bodily response to desires she has hidden away; desires to feel and experience life freely, which she had pushed away out of a need to remain 'dead' for her mother, who never wanted her and tried to abort her. Through her analysis she comes to see her words, her ability to speak of every aspect of her experience, as curative, and to recognise the patriarchal and colonial constraints on her sense of self. She finds a language to talk about her own mother's madness. She recovers – and the bleeding stops.

Before my own experience on the couch, that book had been my gateway into the curative possibility of psychoanalysis – until I read it I had only been able to imagine what went on within the walls of my father's work. It showed me how words and language could release us from tyrannical feelings; and that what we feel in our bodies, what our bodies do, might be mental as well as biological, in ways that we don't consciously know. It made me feel I might one day understand my own trace of bodily clues: the stomach aches I got when I slept at a friend's house; and the headaches that forced me to come home early from parties, the *funeral in my brain* that Emily Dickinson wrote of. Joni had had to learn that poem for an eisteddfod when I was twelve and she was fourteen. I had watched her rehearse, stomp around her bedroom enunciating dramatically – *a service, like a drum / kept beating beating* – and it had stayed in my mind all those years, waiting, perhaps, for me to realise it as an articulation of a dread I came to know too well. The private room of the psychoanalytic setting, where you could say anything at all, was a space I longed for and also feared. Who might I be if I said exactly what I thought?

The answer came when I started seeing Dr Parkes.

My first year in Melbourne I had been alive, euphoric. I had fallen in love both with Gideon and with the city. We moved in together into a small terrace house in Fitzroy, spent our weekends cycling to the city along the river, drinking beer in the sun; we slept curled into each other. We went to bands whenever we could: rock and folk and electronica, learning each other's tastes. We lay in a tent at a music festival listening to the sound of crashing thunder and the strings of the Dirty Three dipping soft and loud in the electric air. He came with me to review plays that were so bad we cried with laughter on the way home. I was back at university studying writing, and in the evenings after class he would be waiting for me in his car, a near-dead Hillman Minx that he bought from a friend. We never let go, holding hands across its cracked-leather bench seat.

And then slowly, anxiety had come again. Nights of recurrent spider dreams, in which I was paralysed by the bite of a poisonous creature that pursued me and attached to me; I got used to feeling exhausted despite apparently sleeping. I got used to irrational thoughts of death and abandonment; that if I didn't hear from Gideon something bad had happened to him. The ghost of my father's mid-marriage revelation haunted me: underneath love there always ran the chance of its severance. I was still a child in mind: I hadn't left my mother at all, only transferred her into Gideon, a new person whom I could never leave.

I had become used to feeling inexplicable nausea whenever the world beckoned beyond my house; parties and dinners and arrangements with friends during which I longed to be back in the quiet of my bedroom. I did not feel safe to grow up after all. The spider that trailed me was adulthood; I had transformed it into a deathly poison that would take me from safety.

Twice a week I went to Dr Parkes's rooms and lay on the couch and tried to say whatever came to me, and cried and laughed and was silent, and listened to him and argued with him. I lay on the couch and hated him and loved him and felt indifferent to him. I lay on the couch and wished I was somewhere else, cringed over what I had to say. I longed for my appointment some weeks and dreaded it others. I always felt better after seeing him. Every time he went away, took a break, the spider dreams returned and the headaches increased and my sadness returned. I brought everything that went through my head, and we kept, together, weaving it into some kind of meaning that I could walk away with and understand, and use to change. He pointed out ways that I repeated behaviours that brought me no gain. Repetition compulsion, Freud called this. The ways we bang our heads against the same walls again and again but seem to not want to. In Freudian terms, the way our defences rise up to protect our unconscious motivations – until we come to understand those motivations and consciously put a stop to them. An analyst does not offer a shoulder to cry on, but asks why on earth we acted the way we did if it brought about such pain.

Five years later I felt ready to face adulthood, ready to be a mother.

Now, again, my knowledge that I was not managing so well came to me when I took stock of how limited living had become: it came in hearing about other mothers doing things I felt unable to do – walking in and out of shops with their baby, and going to the gym and leaving their baby at the creche, and taking their baby to the cinema. Even routine appointments with the maternal and child health nurse felt impossible, and I almost always asked my mother-in-law to come along for support. What exactly I needed support with was unclear even to me, but it ran somewhere along the lines of simply navigating the world. Nothing at all seemed achievable in my fantasies: not breastfeeding in public or changing a nappy away from my home change-table set-up, or finding my way to a given address. And yet, I did every one of these things without fault. The problem lay in the terrible voice in my head that dragged me down and exhausted me with its relentless taunting of what could go wrong.

And it came in instinctively knowing that putting a timetable on Reuben's sleep was a clear overriding of his actual needs. I had read Alice Miller's famous psychoanalytic take on childhood trauma *The Drama of the Gifted Child*: 'Every child has a legitimate need to be noticed, understood, taken seriously, and respected by his mother … the mother gazes at the baby in her arms, and the baby gazes at his mother's face and finds himself therein … provided that the mother is really looking at the unique, small, helpless being and not projecting her own expectations, fears, and plans for the child.'[15] Was I really looking at my baby?

It also came in fleeting realisations of the deprivations I was setting upon myself; in the shrinking of my world. River bike-rides, music, tents, Gideon's body – these were all things belonging to another realm. Mostly, I spent my time at home with Reuben – where I watched him intently or stared out the window at the people passing our house on their way to the train station or to the chemist across the road. Otherwise I walked Reuben in the pram through our suburb, where I could have taken in the cinnamon and clove smells of the shisha-burning cafes, or browsed the Italian supermarket with its ruby bottles of *prosecco* and bulging cheeses. But in those places I felt overwhelmingly vulnerable, the pram always too big or the baby crying too loudly. Instead, I repeated a staid and lonely route past a primary school, the mixed California bungalows and terraces and new townhouses, and back home.

Occasionally I met a friend at a cafe where I tensely watched the clock, and Reuben for signs of displeasure. Otherwise I went to my in-laws', who had moved to a suburb nearby us, and in whose house I felt such warm normality that I was sure no doom could befall me within its walls. There, I spent most of my time staring out their windows, walking Reuben in the pram through their suburb, trying to sleep on their spare bed. I remembered my former life of engaging with literature and eating at restaurants and going to see bands with distant mourning.

My internal state felt like this most of the time: buzzy, jittery, fearful, tense, hyper-alert. I saw disaster in every outcome: my suburban walks were forays into minefields – cars might drive onto the kerb; dogs might lunge at us. The electric snap of a tram line was a live wire coming to get me, and the wasps emerging as spring came were out to sting my baby. At night I only dreamed nightmares: drowning, fires, aeroplane crashes. I was broken, sleepless, stiff from holding my body inert, like a soldier in hiding.

Since that first night in hospital when Gideon had been sent home, I had had a fear of being on my own with Reuben. Really, I feared being on my own with myself. There was no specific event I dreaded – no fantasies of my collapse or of being unable to look after Reuben. It was a fear of having to bear my own dread and panic in the presence of my child. When Gideon had returned to work ten days after Reuben's birth I had stood at the front door sobbing with shock and existential grief. What a naïve dupe I had been: it would be me alone with the baby and my desolate self now for most of our days.

One week Gideon had to go interstate for work for a night. I made it through the first half of the evening alone with Reuben, but just after I had set him back in his cot from a feed, around 2 am, a man – I saw him running away after the fact – inexplicably set off a flare on our front path. The blast and violence of the sound undid me. I wondered if I had conjured this man from my own tenuous mind. I lay awake the rest of the night.

'Make sure you do something nice for yourself each day,' the maternal and child health nurse said to me one visit. 'What do you do that's nice for yourself?' I thought and thought. I thought of the patting and shushing and the time-keeping and the climbing into bed when Gideon came home, and the not being able to read, and the walking the deck in circles. 'I have a cup of coffee,' I told her, and began to cry once more.

In the place of any desire, hunger or living, I had substituted a gaping need for order and predictability, and wishing for that with a small baby in my care was a foolproof route to madness.

At my appointments, I had become filled with rage at Dr Parkes, for his silence, his reticence; for the intermittent scribble of his fountain pen: *Classic resistance*, I imagined him writing (resistance being a form of defence that Freud believed a patient would put up until they were able to incorporate their unconscious motivations into their conscious understanding). For the dizzying cul-de-sac of his interpretations, which insisted on the place that my unconscious was taking in my downfall, on the relationship that went on between us in the room, and which I felt as a silencer of all the very real battles I faced each day: the exhaustion from waking multiple times a night, the oestrogen drops, the pain of my healing body, the unrelenting physical demands of breastfeeding, the loss of my previous freedoms, the stress of caring for another human, the crashing realisation of the inequities of Gideon's and my parental experiences.

Dr Parkes, like all psychoanalysts, focused, in the work we did together, on the dynamics of our relationship, over and above what went on outside the room in which we met – Freud's idea of the *transference*: those strong feelings expressed by the patient about their relationship with the therapist. Contemporary psychoanalysts considered that a person would re-enact with their analyst all their ways of thinking about, their feelings toward and dynamics from their early, formative carers. If you were a baby with a distant, cold mother whom you were always trying to please, you might end up showing this, always acquiescing to what you imagined your analyst's needs to be. You might end up showing somehow that you did not expect your analyst to attend to your needs. And together you might identify this way of being that you had.

But I had become hostile to our work together. Where once I had gained so much from it, even in the intolerable moments of confronting my most ugly feelings, I now found, in my acute panic, only a sense of abandonment in his adherence to always looking at what was going on between us. I needed relief in my world beyond his archaic room with its cornices and glass-doored cabinets and ancient dictionaries.

'You will never, ever understand what it is to have someone rely on your body for their physical survival. I should see a female therapist!' I yelled at him one day. He directed us back to my reliance on him.

'I can't make it. I am sitting in a car full of poo. The baby's nappy exploded,' I cried down the phone one day en route to my appointment. 'You wouldn't understand.' He pointed out that I wanted to explode at him.

And I constantly questioned if my state of crisis was anything more than a reasonable reaction to a trying period of my life.

But I knew that plenty of women faced those same practical battles, and they were able to stop crying. Plenty of women faced those things along with even more challenging realities than mine: poverty, violence, homelessness, disability. We were – all mothers – ground down by the exhaustion, the chaos, the stress, the overwhelming responsibility, and most of us were still, in between it all, eating, and laughing, and seeing friends.

Most significantly, though, I knew that this wasn't the first time I had felt like this: that it had been echoes of these very same feelings that had delivered me to Dr Parkes in the first place, and, if I went further back, to the door of a therapist as a teenager.

6

Maxine had remarried shortly after I'd had the elevator conversation with my father. She met a man who was also from South Africa, and who wielded some power among expats for his business connections. She had gone to meet this man in the hope that he might be able to give her some advice on how to get her children's father into Australia. Aaron and Paul had still been waiting back in South Africa for sponsorships to come through so they could emigrate, and Maxine knew how badly we pined for them. The decision to emigrate to Australia had been a joint one between her and Aaron. Maxine had put aside her devastation and made the divorce amicable, and together they had committed to finding a way for Aaron to be as present as possible in our lives.

While my mother met with this man, Joni and I played on the balcony of his apartment, which looked out to Perth's Swan River. In a few months, we would spend weekends on that river learning to water ski, pulled by his speedboat. He was magnanimous, charismatic.

Their wedding was two years later at a boathouse on the river. My mother was thirty-four. It was a warm summer night and Joni and I wore Thai silk dresses and had our hair crimped. My father and Paul were there: they had both finally made it to Perth, begun to settle in to their new life together in Australia. Joni's and my reunion with them was short-lived: weeks after my mother remarried we left them again, to move to Sydney, where my stepfather had started a new business.

Soon, I saw that my stepfather liked to show off his power. I saw it in the ostentatious house we moved into with him among the mansions of Sydney's North Shore, with its pool and spa and four levels and grand chandelier, and in the way he liked to leave to drop me off at school ten minutes too late, so that I was in a state of tension the whole drive. In the way he talked about his own success and generosity, how many jobs he had given back in South Africa to poor men from the townships, how many business deals he had sealed. And not long after they married, in the way he belittled my mother. She came home from their honeymoon in sunny Thailand looking pale, drawn. Later, when I was an adult, she told me she knew already on that honeymoon that she had made a terrible mistake.

Our household became a wreckage of violent exchanges; nights were punctuated by yelling, accusations, the rise and fall of their voices, sharp, wounding, thunderous. I lay in my bed in the room that shared a wall with theirs and felt adrenalin course through me. In the morning, like on a beach that has survived a tsunami, there were the clues of damage – silences and clenched jaws – and then would come a loving apology from my stepfather, in time for a lavish dinner party for visiting business associates from Japan or China or Switzerland, at which my mother would play dutiful hostess and fill an antique dining table with abundant plates of smoked fish, blue cheese croquettes, bagels, cold pastrami, hot beef. My sister and I would be sent into the room with trays of blinis, bowls of creamed mushroom soup, warm bread rolls.

Confusingly, I loved my stepfather. From when I was nine, he had filled, in a practical way, a significant parental role in my daily life. It was he who danced the waltz with me at my primary school graduation; it was he who shouted from the sidelines at my netball games. He called me his daughter, and he showed affection to me as easily as a father would, holding my hand or putting his arm around me with pride. He did not do this with my sister. Joni was not as good as I was at being the right sort of person for someone else. She was more inclined to have the wrong haircut for girls our age or to bring sullen, odd friends home to watch sci-fi videos in the video machine that my stepfather was using to record the cricket.

Sometimes we were a happy family, enjoying a summer barbecue. Normal family things happened in our house (goldfish were bought and died and accidentally catapulted onto the neighbour's roof instead of into the bushes), and not normal things happened (ledgers of our phone usage were kept and monitored by my stepfather; my mother was often to be found crying in the toilet).

I reached sixteen shell-shocked from the escalating fights. I found conflict of any sort overwhelming, woke every morning with an empty feeling of dread, couldn't stay away from home for sleepovers with friends without waking in the night with fear. I had become my mother's witness. Lodged in me was that growing, but not yet consciously formed, sense of myself: I was conceived of hope for my mother. What I did know was that away from her I had a certainty that catastrophe would strike because of my absence.

Shortly after turning seventeen, I did try to leave Maxine. I signed up for an exchange trip to France, to live in Paris with a woman named Sabine and her two small children for a month, and then with a family in a small village in the south for close to a year. I had wanted to start university in France, but they had strict rules about what age you could study there, and I was told I was not yet old enough. I settled on a high-school exchange in which I would repeat my final year of study but in French, at a school in the south. I had saved some money from the various jobs I had worked at during school, at a photo-printing outlet and babysitting, but the trip itself I could not pay for. My mother paid for it using money she had saved from her own work, which she kept in a secret account separate from my stepfather's riches so she could spend without incurring his wrath.

My school friends threw me a surprise farewell party. It was like a childhood party, rather than the new kind of drunken party everyone was getting into with too many Sub Zeroes and carpets damp with rum and coke. In a well-lit lounge room the boys played on their guitars, and the girls sat around eating crisps. They must have recognised in me already a kind of regression. They were all going off to university or to travel, while I was going back to school.

I was going to miss my friends. We were besotted with each other, bound by the intimacy of high school, the platonic love that comes from suffering through exams and squashy assemblies and crammed school buses together. We wrote each other letters, despite being in each other's company every minute of every weekday. At the party that night we took photos of ourselves in oddly formal poses, like family portraits. I had gotten a sty in my eye that week, and in the photos I look weepy, drained. I was starting to feel the deep regret of being perched on the end of a high diving board with an audience. There was no refund for changing your mind – there was no backing out.

A week later, my mother took me to the airport. I cried the whole way there; it felt as though I was on my way to purgatory rather than to a year of European delights. The moment the aeroplane descended over Paris, the sickening dread bore down on me with force. I thought I might throw up, but gathered myself, shaking and clammy.

Outside the arrival gates a stern blonde woman held up a sign with my name. She did not smile at me. I followed her out into the cold grey Paris air, into her tiny European car. She spoke to me only in French. Seated in her car, she said: 'I am Sabine. You cannot stay with me. My daughter has just broken her arm.' I understood the French but nothing of what she said made sense. I was too tired and too busy trying to hold my body together to ask anything. She took me on a winding, labyrinthine drive through the centre of Paris, blanketed in fog and now getting dark. I was sure I was in hell.

At her apartment, I passed out on her couch, where I woke some hours later utterly confused and ill with jetlag. A man and a woman loomed above me, both wearing those too-square aviator glasses that give people the look of a serial killer. 'We are taking you to a friend who can have you stay,' they told me in French. I had no idea who they were, or where they were taking me. I wasn't sure anymore if I was feeling irrational fear or real external threat; perhaps I was about to be murdered after all. I asked if I could phone home, and Sabine handed me her house phone. I tried to explain to my mother what was going on, but I had no idea myself, and in any case it wasn't the logistical sequence of broken arms or swapped hosts that I needed to tell her about; there were no words for this thing inside me.

The serial killers escorted me to their tiny European car, and for an age we wended our way through more darkened streets, following the dim yellow streak of their fog lights. I hadn't eaten in more than a day, but my stomach had closed up in any case.

At last, we arrived at a house in the suburban outskirts of Paris, where the man and the woman deposited me and my giant suitcase in the mud at the front door and rang the bell. A small, bright-eyed woman opened it and ordered me in French to take off my boots. Then she saw me in. The fear that I felt then, in removing the shoes that had clung to me since home, the culture shock – it coalesced into something like vertigo. It was dark, and I could see no further than a small forest of fir trees beside the house. Both within my body and beyond the borders of my skin I had arrived at a hostile, strange place. I could not go back home – my mother had paid for this trip with her hard-earned secret money.

I sat at that kitchen table, shaking, unable to talk, trying to follow the rapid French that the man and woman were spitting out. Two raggedly beautiful children ran around the four of us, playing. Shortly, the man and woman left and I could hold myself together no more.

Ψ

The bright-eyed woman's name was Melanie. She spoke English with the most glorious lilting Irish accent. 'I will get you someting to feel better,' she said to me. 'And I will phone your mother.'

She left the room. The children stared at me with curiosity. '*Salut*,' I ventured in a wobbly voice. I tried to calm my breathing. The house smelled of washing powder and faintly of cigarettes.

Melanie returned with the phone, and I called my mother again. This time I assured her I was okay, which was to say I was no longer in imminent danger of being sliced up by unfashionable French serial killers. I passed the phone to Melanie, who spoke gently and with assurance. 'She will stay here with us now,' she said.

Off the phone, she handed me a small tablet. 'Your mother says you can take this. It will calm you.' I took it, whatever it was, and ate some of the macaroni and cheese she had made for the children, and let her make me a cup of chamomile *tisane*, which I sipped slowly while she bathed the children and got them to bed.

Soon after, her husband, Francois, a quiet philosophy teacher who quickly revealed himself to be the source of the cigarette smell, arrived home and Melanie briefed him on the profusely swallowing Australian basket-case seated at his kitchen table.

After that, they filled me in on how I had ended up in their care. Melanie and Francois had started taking students in through the exchange program, and now they had received this call. Yes, Sabine's daughter had broken her arm. But also, Sabine's husband had killed himself not long before I arrived, and at some point, perhaps when I was in the air over Bahrain brewing my panic, she had decided it was a bad idea to house a stranger. I seemed always to be on-call as an understudy for absent husbands.

Since the pill and the *tisane* had begun to sedate me, I was relatively unperturbed by this new plot twist, merely grateful to have been taken in to the maternal bosom of people who seemed to treat seriously that I was sliding into my own private catastrophe. In any case, I was rapidly becoming near-catatonic, and soon collapsed into the bed they had made up for me, shivering uncontrollably into a deep sleep, despite long-johns, a tracksuit and a heavy duvet.

At 3 am my eyes snapped open and the terror began to unspool in me again. *I am too far from home*, I thought. My pulse raced, my skin tingled, my whole body shook. I put the light on and was enveloped by the strange physical dislocation of jetlag: the hunger of morning felt fiercely in a night-times' darkness; the sense, in the deep silence of 3 am, that birds should be singing. I had nothing to distract myself; the books on the shelf were all Francois' French philosophy texts, and I was not bearing the faculties to conjugate foreign verbs. I moved in and out of my own body in a dream state of half-sleep, up into the freezing Paris air like a ghost, high as the Eiffel Tower; but never could I get myself above the fog, to conjure a feeling that I was still connected with home, that in fact an aeroplane could take me back should I wish to return. I felt I was completely cut off from my mother in a dangerous way; that this decision to come to Paris, this city of too-adult things like romance and heady cheeses and wine, meant that I would never again be able to return to the safety of her body.

7

I came home after only six weeks in France. The month in Paris with Melanie and Francois had passed somehow. Francois had driven me to the train station every morning in the freezing dark to get the metro into the city to sit in a small, windowless room with other English-speaking students, where we went over conversational French for hours. In the Paris shops, the salespeople spoke back to me in English. Perhaps they sensed how stricken I was, how on the edge; that I needed language that would hold me.

I had thought I might be able to ride out my internal terror in the company of understanding people; that maybe it was culture shock. So Melanie put in a request that I stay the rest of the year with them and attend school in Paris instead of moving on to the family in the south. But the program managers came back with a curt response: '*Non.*'

I went to the seaside village with heavy reluctance. The new family who received me, unable to understand this wreck of an Australian girl, were unsympathetic to my state. '*Le mal du pays!*' the father exclaimed. Homesickness, nothing more.

They had in place a series of punitive rules that, in my precarious state, caused me to lie awake at night in their vast castle and wonder if I was involved in a people-trafficking ring: I was not to use their phone, and they asked to keep my passport. It was so hard to separate out real threat from my mind's looping reign of terror. I refused to give them my passport.

Daily, I went off to school, trailing behind the daughters – who remained impassive to my presence – to the bus stop, where I sat between raucous French adolescents who reeked of Gauloises and ignored me. It suited me to be ignored; I was atomising, breaking up into tiny particles. I couldn't possibly exist and attempt French conversation at the same time.

In the second week with them, exhausted from the effort of reminding myself I wasn't dying, I made a decision to go home. Released from the fantasy of my own imminent demise I ate all the chocolate-covered macadamia nuts I had brought over in gift boxes as thank-yous to future friends and then, in some kind of sugar euphoria, going against house rules, I ordered a cab from their phone, dragged my heavy suitcase down the cobblestone driveway and escaped back to Paris, to Melanie and Francois, and a few days later to London, to where I had pleaded with my mother to come. There, at a hotel in Belsize Park, I fell into the crook of her arm, defeated.

Revival by chocolate was not an overstatement. Because, first, before the trip to France, there had been another problem. This one was as much to do with my body as my mind. My body had become alarmingly thin. I hadn't meant for it to. On a day in September, a few months before the fateful trip to France, the weather inching toward summer with dips and lurches of Sydney's tropical heat and humidity, I had received photos in the mail from the French host family in the south: the girls of the family were lithe, skiing effortlessly down slopes on rake-thin legs. I had wanted to fit into that family. I wanted to fit into the figure of a girl who belonged in a happy family that went on joyful ski holidays. Not like the holiday we had recently been on that had ended in an apartment on the Gold Coast with my mother and stepfather locked in another dangerous conflict. I had taken a school friend with me for that holiday. We had sat in the back of the car, trapped in the simmering adult tension, from Sydney to the Gold Coast. My friend had gotten so carsick we had had to stop numerous times for her to vomit. I was mortified at the catastrophe that holiday had become. In a kind of self-punishment I had chopped all my hair off. At school, the boys wanted to know why I had cut my hair like a man. It was a year of feeling I wanted to disappear.

And the school formal was coming up. I decided to lose a few kilos. I'd do it with extra exercise and by cutting out fat. It would be easy. I could swim laps of our pool, set at the bottom of our garden.

I began to prepare my own school lunch instead of letting my mother do it: a small container of rice mixed with pumpkin. I knew about calorie counting and fat grams: we'd had a Weight Watchers meal plan booklet in our house since I was seven when my mother, in hindsight inexplicably, sent Joni to a meeting. My sister was not fat. I was not fat either. I had been athletic as a child; I'd watched Zola Budd on television break world records at the Olympics in bare feet and I had practised running on the spot until my heels pounded. Joni and I had become women young, no longer fitting into children's wear past the age of ten on account of hips and breasts. I lived in dread of the *Plotkin legs*, as my mother called them: the thick ankles and chunky thighs of my Eastern European ancestors. I decided when I was five that I did indeed have fat knees. When I was eight, living in Perth, where summers were spent in bathers, I wrote in my diary that I was going on a diet. I never stayed on them, but my notebooks were speckled with attempts to keep track of my food intake, with resolutions for healthier eating, with *perfect body* plans torn out from magazines. Growing up, then in Sydney with my mother and stepfather and sister, diets were always spoken about: my stepfather had high cholesterol, and my mother made it her mission to lower it. But he also had a ravenous appetite – for Kettle chips, bagels, pastrami; and for the foods of his childhood, procured from South African visitors or a local South African food supplier: *biltong* (dried jerky), *mebos* (a flattened preserve made from dried fruits). Temptation was everywhere, snuck away in his study desk; hidden in the trick drawer of the antique armoire in the third, and most formal, lounge.

This time, I was as studious with my diet as I was with the final exams I was revising for, for which I scribbled out ten practice essays a day. Mornings before school I churned eighty laps of our swimming pool, lines from my English papers pounding the beat of my strokes. Graham Greene and Charles Dickens. Gerard Manly Hopkins: *Not, I'll not, carrion comfort, Despair, not feast on thee;/ Not untwist – slack they may be – these last strands of man/ In me or, most weary, cry I can no more. I can.* After that, I ate a bowl of Special K with two tablespoons of skim milk. Then I ate an apple at recess, my rice and pumpkin at lunch, a fat-free yoghurt after school and the vegetable component of whatever dinner my mother had prepared. The weight dropped off me. I felt elated. I went to sleep at night going over a list of what I had consumed: it quietened the noise of the fighting from the room next door. I started waking earlier and earlier, doing more and more laps, now listing fewer and fewer items consumed as I fell asleep. I stood in front of the open fridge late at night and observed, with a proud sense of my steely will, all the food I no longer ate: cheeses, cold meats, mayonnaise, juice, salad dressing, chocolate, butter. Nothing mattered now: not the perilous state of my home life or the question of my mother's survival or the adrenalin from hearing the shouting. With each kilo dropped I felt a peaceful numbness settle over me. An invincibility.

The end of the year, and adult independence, loomed, and I awaited it with equal excitement and dread. I wrote in my diary that I wanted to be small again. A little girl.

When my exam results came through I had gotten a high enough score to study Law. I had come second in the state for English. And I had lost ten kilos. I was thin enough to go to France.

I went to my school formal in an ice-blue corseted floor-length gown, my waist cinched tight. I was Cinderella at the ball: a mere glass slipper away from adulthood. In photos it looks like a wedding dress. The boy I took to the formal, the unsuitable first love, was utterly unavailable to me, always bringing other girls along on our dates or leaving me waiting. I wrote in my diary as I cried over him: *I am always trying to get my father back.*

Failure to thrive. That's what my trip to France was. I had tried to leave home and I couldn't. I could no longer ignore the taut rope that yanked me back to the safety of my mother.

On the surface of things, I now began my life as a young adult: I started an Arts/Law degree, and upped my career stakes from the cashier jobs I'd held after taking a flyer from the law school noticeboard to try out to be trained as an editor for a legal publisher. But I had performed some kind of magic and doubled myself: a simulacrum with no desire or appetite or beating heart set off each day on the train to class, where the words of the lecturers bounced off my robot self. On my notepad, I formed the motions of note-taking, but mostly I tallied my day's food intake. When exam time came I made up for my in-class fugue state by studying with the tenacity I applied to my dieting, and somehow I continued to pass. I went to parties, and drank, and smoked, and watched with detached interest as my girl friends partnered off with the well-bred private-school boys that already spoke with the performative confidence of barristers.

My heart had been broken by the few unsuitable boys I had chosen to focus on since France. Physical intimacy never led to the emotional intimacy I was after; the connection that would assure me of love, of them staying, not leaving. No man had proved to be as attached to me as I had been to him. The pain separation caused me made casual relationships, burgeoning relationships, on-and-off relationships – of which my and my friends' lives substantially centred on – unbearable. Though I put on a good show of being the kind of girl who sweated the night away at raves, wedged between fluorescent-panted young men, the kind who head-banged with abandon in the close, steamy confines of testosterone-filled grunge gigs, I was ill-suited to the life of a young woman in late-'90s Australia, where frivolous fun and fleeting connections, one-night-stands and flirtation were the norm. I would have been perfect for a nineteenth-century novel, uncomfortably perched on my settee, prevented from prostrating myself in grief only by a stiff bustle, waiting for my one true love. I almost always regretted going out, wishing I had instead stayed on my own at home, reading.

Now my heart was metal. I studiously avoided a reciprocated relationship. Once, a quiet, gentle guy from my sociology class followed me out to the walkway when I left a seminar early. He handed me a note and scuttled off. It said: *My name is Josh. I think you seem really nice. If you would like to have a coffee, here is my number.* I threw the piece of paper away and never went back to sociology.

There glimmered at the edge of my vision the joy of English, which was my Arts degree major, but my frozen state could not accommodate real, lived pleasure. It was hard to read when you were starving. Another me was back home in my mother's bed.

And my mother's bed did indeed now have a space vacated for me. My stepfather had crossed the threshold of psychological abuse: 'He hit me,' my mother told me, sobbing in Joni's old bedroom, a few weeks before I realised home was now sitting on a faultline and made my own escape to Joni's dingy apartment overlooking a petrol station. The morning after his transgression, Joni and I helped Maxine transport whatever we could fit of hers into her car to pile it into a house she and my stepfather had bought and were about to move into. A lawyer had advised my mother to stake her claim on it by taking occupation. For a decade I dreamed, in vivid detail, the contents of the childhood bedroom I had hastily packed up in those weeks of familial disintegration. Mostly I dreamed there was a cupboard I had forgotten to look in that contained all my precious items: my jewellery box, my tin with letters from my father.

I never saw my stepfather again, aside from one unfortunate crossing of paths with him at a party of a friend whose parents knew him, where the grief of losing him – even despite his reign of terror – melded with the grief of my father leaving, such that I was overcome by a depth of crying that bordered on hysteria. My ambivalence toward him, along with loyalty to my mother, who had been traumatised by the emotional violence of their marriage, meant that I was never able to resolve an ending with him. It was as though he had died but could not be mourned.

Bodily, I was on a fast rewind back to infancy. By the end of that year, I had lost another five kilos. Now without access to a pool, I joined a gym. Exercise was about elimination. At first, an aerobics class felt good enough to balance out whatever I had eaten. But soon that wasn't enough to get the numb elation of thinness. I would run on the treadmill for half an hour, then do the aerobics class. If I skipped a day at the gym, if I ate a piece of toast, I was certain that I was huge and became overwhelmed with self-hatred and hopelessness. I went away to the coast with a group of friends and watched as they ate kebabs and burgers, drank beer and stuffed their faces with chips, lay on the sand and baked their still slim but satiated bodies. Why could I not eat those things and stay thin? Why did eating one hot chip make me feel so bleak and blown-out that I had to punish myself by eating nothing the next day? My mind had grown warped. I couldn't see that I was too thin. I looked at my bony arms and legs and saw heft. I knew I was on a slippery slope: I had forgotten how to eat to give my body the right amount of energy. If I ate an apple my stomach bloated and I was certain I was fat. I was in an impossible bind. I couldn't eat at all or I would keep gaining, keep gaining. But if I didn't eat at all I would die. I didn't want to die; I just wanted the thin-euphoria that made nothing else matter. The group went out for a friend's breakfast and I watched them all eating bacon and eggs and felt paralysed by my inability to choose a food from the menu. I left the group to find a phone box and called my mother. 'I need help,' I said to her.

And so I arrived at my first therapist, waif-like and stuck. He was a gently spoken Indian man, a practising Buddhist. Into his rooms spilled a clear light from floor-to-ceiling windows. The train line ran along beside us, the rhythmic *thunk thunk* and then *toot* of express services filling my silences. I sat on a grey leather couch that faced him. I found it hard to look him in the eye. My father paid for my sessions, and I accepted his help. I needed it.

The therapist showed me warmth. 'I am so proud of you,' he said, when I told him my poetry was going to be published. He put me onto medication: an antidepressant. He said that the dieting was a response to anxiety and depression. 'You are in crisis. You want to be nourished,' he told me, when I began seeing him and explained the shards of my home life, how I missed my father back in Perth, my gruelling food regimen. Again that not-line between my mind and my flesh. And he was right, in a literal sense. I was trying to get my mother's attention with my frailty – I was trying to get her to tend to me rather than to the drama of her marriage. He gave me that parental attention. He gave me his phone number. I could ring him if I needed to, he told me. And I did. For years I rang him; one year, when I was twenty-one and took a break from study to backpack around Europe and the Middle East, I rang him every week from a phone box. His wife usually answered the phone. I would need to hear his voice, to fill in the gaping nothingness that threatened to replace my calorie counting. He gave me articles to read on meditation, and cassette tapes of him leading guided journeys. I saw him twice a week for six years, with that year overseas in among it all. That trip was the only time I had been able to go away from home and not experience that fall into anxiety. Why was that time different to my France trip? Perhaps I felt the Buddhist therapist was travelling with me; perhaps it was because I was travelling with a close friend who stood in for home. Or perhaps it was simply that I was on the antidepressants, boxes of which were taking up a good quarter of the precious little space I had in my backpack.

In those six years, I finished my Law degree, and I gained all the weight back. On our last session together I brought him a box of chocolates and he opened it and we shared them. As a parting gift he gave me a copy of Winnicott's seminal book *Playing and Reality*. In it he wrote: *May you continue to play and enjoy the reality of fully living.* Later that final year with him, with my studies completed and a burgeoning return of good feeling, I took myself off medication and moved to Melbourne. I left my mother.

8

I thought a lot about the Buddhist therapist now. I googled him and felt a kick of grief, seeing his familiar, gentle face again and remembering how he had expressed kindness to me. *You* are *a good person*, he would tell me, apropos of nothing, in the space at the end of a session when I had nothing to say. I could conjure his voice in my head still. Sometimes at night when I lay on the floor of Reuben's room watching the red light of the baby monitor blinking, I summoned it to lead me on a meditation, as he did in the tapes he had given me. *Relax. Find yourself a calm space for quiet and solitude to do these exercises*, he always began. Under the baby's cot seemed to meet those criteria.

The Buddhist therapist was not a psychoanalyst, but a psychodynamic therapist, like my father, working with his patients by considering their unconscious mental lives but with less adherence to Freudian technique. He was not far off a Freudian interpretation of my self-imposed starvation when he said I was reaching for babyhood again. Freud understood appetite as an expression of a person's life instinct or libido. Starvation in adolescence, Freud said, was a way of repressing sexual maturity; a way to stop the body maturing into adulthood, and to stop a separation from the mother. Perhaps it was no coincidence that I had launched myself into this state of self-starvation right as I stood on the precipice of school-leaving, of adulthood. I wasn't ready to leave my mother.

That her survival depended on me was not a conscious thought

I had but an undercurrent of feeling in me that had grown more urgent with the escalating violence of her marriage. To some extent the Buddhist therapist came to this understanding of me by paying attention to what I was expressing unknowingly, in my voice, my words, my body, but he worked far more on the surface of things than a psychoanalyst might, possibly because he sensed that I needed care at that point more than I needed to understand myself. He paid much less attention to the transference, the way that how I related to him might shed light on my problem. He did not try to be neutral in his responses to me, which Freud had seen as necessary for the transference to occur. Our mission, it seemed, was to rebuild my sense of worth, attend to my self-esteem, halt my obsessive eating pattern, and to do so he went out of his way to offer me words that were the opposite of neutral, that were deliberately paternal and loving – *You* are *worthwhile*, he would say to me – in worksheets he gave me to take home, in the group sessions he ran, where many of his patients would gather together in a room to meditate and undertake exercises to improve their self-confidence.

Later, when I was in psychoanalysis with Dr Parkes, these exercises and surface interpretations felt trite, but I often yearned for them. I saw that the kind of work I did with Dr Parkes was more about knowing and self-sufficiency: at worst a dire existential exercise, at best a hopeful creative act. What use would it be to spend more years patching up where the cracks were by using the putty of another person's positive affirmation and kindness? Psychoanalysis with Dr Parkes served the purpose of an engineering surveyor: it felt out the cause of the cracks to begin with.

But now, I needed to talk through whether it was reasonable to wait out finding the cracks; whether that kind of work could be helpful to me in such a state of crisis. The Buddhist therapist was the perfect sounding board for this question. I flew back to Sydney with six-month-old Reuben for a week.

Ψ

Donald Winnicott suggested that Freud had intuitively chosen for the analytic setting an environment and set of conditions that evoked early childhood for the patient, so that they would regress and more easily reveal their infantile fantasies. Among these features, Winnicott included that: 'This work was to be done in a room, not a passage, a room that was quiet and not liable to sudden unpredictable sounds, yet not dead quiet and not free from ordinary house noises. The room would be lit properly, not by a light staring into the face, and not by a variable light. The room would certainly not be dark and it would be comfortably warm. The patient would be lying on a couch, that is to say comfortable if able to be comfortable, and probably a rug and some water would be available.'[16]

Dr Parkes's consulting rooms adhered almost identically to that description. They were attached to his house. I would hear a person I assumed to be his wife padding up and down a hallway on the other side of the wall beside me, and a door creaking open and shut, sometimes a woman's voice. The room itself was dim, textural, opulent in its aesthetic: ox-blood, oak, velvet, paisley, fabric-covered books, rugs, a soft light from a cream lantern, and always a flower in a state of undress, or death, losing its petals on a side table.

There were so many entrances to get to the inner room where the work was done. First, a gate from the street that opened into a small garden where you rang a brass bell that sat on a small wooden table and waited. A click sounded and released a door that opened onto a waiting room. I never encountered another of Dr Parkes's patients. His waiting room was for one person; a sort of decompression chamber before entering the room where the work would be done. This suited me. I found it shameful to be seen entering therapy.

The waiting room had three doors, including the entrance. One, always slightly ajar, led to a small washroom. One led to the consulting room. That door was the most curious. It had a bottom half that opened separately from the top half. You had to open the top, and then you could open the bottom. Was it to allow the process of leaving to happen slowly? They confounded me always, those two part-doors.

The very first time I had gone to see Dr Parkes I had waited in a wicker chair in the waiting room until the split doors had opened and a man had stepped out into the waiting area. I'd wanted to smile. He looked like Freud.

In the consulting room I'd stood awkwardly, unsure of where to go. Dr Parkes had watched me. I saw the couch, one that looked like Freud's famous chaise longue. I wasn't ready for that. I'd sat in an armchair that was set up opposite another armchair. He'd taken a seat in the other one.

A few weeks later I'd summoned the courage to lie on the couch, thinking I was finally a good patient, doing proper analysis. I'd battled with this feeling of being good and then bad, moving from couch to chair, until one day I had realised there was no right or wrong in that room and that I was free to choose.

The Buddhist therapist, on the other hand, was part of a bustling joint practice and had a receptionist and a waiting room full of people reading magazines. I hid behind a magazine, remembering how in my six years of seeing him I had burned with embarrassment at being in that room with the other patients and felt it was inherently wrong to be made to come face to face with strangers in that context. After a session, my eyes would be puffy from crying, my breath shuddery. I would keep my head down and scuttle out the building, terrified I might see someone I knew, see my child-self watching at the window like I used to do at my father's house where he saw his patients. And the group sessions – I had gone to a few but I had felt overwhelmingly self-conscious, and worried there was something distasteful about acknowledging that we all saw the same therapist. Something that broke boundaries and inclined us toward worshipping him.

Now, after seven years, the Buddhist therapist opened his door and called me in brightly, embracing me as I crossed the threshold into his rooms. *Dr Parkes would never hug me,* I thought. The room seemed garishly upholstered and light. I sat on the couch facing him, unable to find a comfortable position amid its pouffy rainbow cushions. *This is awkward,* I thought, recalling the simple ease of Dr Parkes's firm upholstery. He smiled and congratulated me on becoming a mother. *Dr Parkes had been careful not to congratulate me, lest he make assumptions about how I was experiencing motherhood and prevent me expressing myself fully,* I remembered.

I told him about the sleep tallies, and the tumbling thoughts and the panic, about the dread each day and the way I felt when Reuben cried. I told him how I wasn't writing or reading or cooking. And I told him the details of how I had come to see Dr Parkes years before. Seeing Dr Parkes had helped me, I told him.

'You speak so positively about your analysis,' he said to me as our time drew to a close. 'I can hear you value it. But you may need something more right now.' His offerings were always like fortune-cookie notes.

I was not yet convinced of what exactly I did need, but I would be within a few days. Maxine flew back with us to Melbourne – 'I'm worried about you,' she said – and we agreed she would stay a few days.

On the second day we decided to go to a shopping centre. I had not done anything so ordinary since before Reuben was born, all such gratuitous activities having left the realm of my considerations. But Maxine convinced me that it would be good to venture out, maybe buy myself some new clothes. She had been coming to spend time with us every month or so. She stayed in our spare room, filling the house with items I had long connected with her presence: a radio beside the bed that she told me she could not sleep without, from which blared talkback, and which I had come to understand was her way of keeping thoughts out of her head in the loneliness of night; empty teacups, burned toast left in the toaster to be eaten at midnight when she required a dose of insulin and food, an accumulation of newly purchased domestic props she had identified as lacking in my house – roll-a-towel, dishwashing liquid, a banana hanger.

I still hadn't been able to broach with her how devastating the timing of her sudden departure had been for me in those first weeks of motherhood. I had folded away into myself my anger and disappointment with her for having put her own conflict with my father front and centre then. I knew that watching me come home with my husband and new baby must have revived difficult feelings for her. But I couldn't understand what caused her to feel so furious or powerless that not being there to support me had seemed like a better idea than staying and bearing her own pain.

I was so grateful to have her there now – for, although we fought, she mercilessly made me laugh. She saw absurdity in everything: 'Why,' she deadpanned one evening while visiting, as we watched a news clip about renovations at the zoo, 'would a grown adult wave at an animal?' On the television a middle-aged woman was smiling vacantly and flapping her hand at a lemur.

And of course the presence of another adult was what I craved then, for it alleviated my fear of what might happen to Reuben if I became incapacitated by my own panic. I avoided raising the spectre of her having left when I needed her most in case it caused her to leave again; in my perilous state I was not sure I could survive that.

So I strapped Reuben in the car, bolstered by her presence, sure that I could again find it in myself to enjoy the superficial comforts of consumerism. My mother and I had always had our best times in shopping centres. Our glory days had been spent escalator-riding and trying on clothes and finally collapsing into the booth of a linoleum-seated cafe with our purchases to revive ourselves on toasted asparagus and cheese sandwiches under a jaundiced fluorescent light. We were at our best when we could snicker together at the absurdities of other people from behind a shopfront awning.

The shopping centre was as little as five kilometres from the house, and I had driven there a few times over the years. It was an easy route – straight down a main road and a few lefts and rights. But now, where to turn? The street was longer than I remembered. Unrecognisable. Why weren't there signs on every corner? People drove too fast. Had I left the oven on? Wait – I was thinking of another shopping centre. Reuben squawked; I sweated. I took us around in circles; my knuckles grew white on the steering wheel. I stopped twice, three times to consult my GPS. I wound down the window to let in air. Reuben cried; I made a high-pitched squeak that I had never heard myself make before and quickly realised it was a prelude to my own crying. My mother told me to calm down. I pulled over and put my head on the steering wheel – why was this so hard? When had living become so impossible? I turned the car around and drove us home, defeated.

Later, with Reuben asleep and my mother in bed, I confided in Gideon. 'I'm not doing that well.'

'No kidding,' he said, half-smiling.

I phoned my father. 'I need the name of a psychiatrist.'

9

Maternal separation had long preoccupied me, but it was only after Reuben was born that I felt the cyclical implications of being both mother and child. I considered my own belly button with confusion, as though I had never encountered it. What did it represent – was it where I was attached to my mother or where I was attached to my son? Something in the physical experience of becoming a mother had tangled my lifelines. When the tiny bloodied stumps of umbilical cord fell off the soft bellies of both my sons I felt unexpected grief: there lay the rampart between us, and I felt I was to spend the next life re-imagining it in a bid to keep them safe, those bodies that I had grown.

Perhaps the confusion lay in my sense that Joni and I had a part in keeping my mother safe. We had been her companions since Aaron left.

'What kind of mother are you, bringing your children to this movie?' a woman once barked at Maxine in the dark of the cinema in the year we emigrated to Australia. She had taken Joni and me along with her to see the Bette Midler and Danny DeVito movie *Ruthless People*, about a man who is ecstatic when his overbearing wife is kidnapped. We were too young for that movie, and maybe Maxine made an error of judgement taking us. But she was thirty-three years old, on her own in a new country, without any family. There were always reasons we were compelled to stay together, Maxine, Joni and me.

I had felt the pull of her need for us before then, already.

In the drive to the video store, where she would stock up on bags of movies to tide the weekend over, I'd felt it. At home, when the credits rolled and the cartoons were over, I'd felt it. I would wake at night and feel an urgent need to go to her bed. There was room for me, because Aaron wasn't there. It took just the right quiet midnight circumstances – the muted light of the passageway, that untenably loud radio which was always beside her – to know the loss their separation represented for her.

I felt, too, Aaron's absence from her side in the ways that Joni and I assumed roles of care for her that my father might have if he had been there. I knew of the real, physiological threat to herself that my mother's body carried, in the form of her diabetes, in ways that might have been buffered by the presence of a father. I saw her inject her thigh every few hours, knew that the black box she wore on a belt around her waist had a long, thin tube with a needle at one end that went into her abdomen, carrying the strangely antiseptic-smelling liquid that her body needed to stay alive. And how much she hated wearing it, which she told me.

Late one night when I was four, climbing into her bed, I saw her try to reach for the phone on the bedside table. Her hand seemed claw-like, rigid. I watched as she struggled to reach the cord and then rolled off the bed, hitting the floor hard. I ran back to the room I shared with Joni. 'Mom is sick!' I shouted. Joni knew what to do: she went to the pantry and gave her a jar of honey. My mother stuck her hand into the jar like bears I had seen pawing honey out of hives on nature documentaries, scooping it into her mouth until she seemed herself again. Joni and I did the right thing, she told us. We were so brave and clever. My mother's hand was shredded from the glass jar, long cuts running down her thumb and outer palm. After that night I started having a recurring nightmare that she was standing on a street corner leaking fluid from her stomach, dying, and that I was beside her but unable to do anything. Then, when I was an adult, Maxine nearly slipped into unconsciousness three times through low blood-sugar and it was me who found her, or me whom she reached out to. One of those times we were nine hundred kilometres apart. I was trying on my wedding dress in a change room in the city in Melbourne and she was in her bedroom in Sydney. It was my final dress fitting. My phone kept ringing – it was Maxine. But every time I answered it there was no one on the other end. It rang, it rang, it rang, it rang. Joni still lived in Sydney so I phoned her. She also tried Maxine, to no avail. 'I'm driving over there,' she told me.

'Don't cry! You'll stain the dress!' the seamstress warned me. But I couldn't stop – what would Joni find? Maxine became furious with me when she found out how much I had panicked about her health. 'It's happened many more times when you've known nothing about it, and I am always fine,' she told me. But my dreams. The idea of her death, and my helplessness beside her, was too far inside me.

When my stepfather showed that he would abscond from loving her too, I again felt a compulsion to fill the void of absent fathers, and a fear that if I did not she might not survive. The fear overwhelmed me at many points in my life when I was at a symbolic or actual great distance from her, a long time before France, sometimes so insidiously that I wasn't even aware of its connection to the events of my life. It came when I was reaching the middle of high school, when I had begun to relish the independence of going into the city on my own on the train, taking in the lush suburbia of Sydney, the voyeurism of watching strangers in the window reflection in the tunnels, the serendipity of walking without a plan through its streets and arcades. It thrashed down on me, a shape-shifter: soon after that enjoyment, I no longer felt okay at school, which was a long way from home on the other side of Sydney. What were regular if unpleasant experiences of schoolyard conflict at my all-girls school, mean note-passing and name-calling and ganging up, became unbearable for me: I would wake with nausea, dread, a sense that I might die. At the end of that year, I decided to leave the school I had once loved, to go to a different one. Later, I realised, the new school I chose was by design closer to my mother. That perhaps the schoolyard conflict had had little bearing on my terror. And it happened again when I went on a holiday camp for the first time: the nausea was so bad that I was given a quiet, dark room to lie in, suspected of gastro. It improved once I had made it through the first night away, awake and plotting how I might walk back through the thickets of bush we had arrived at by bus, but never lifted until I was home.

In my choice of literature I tested out our mutual leaving of each other. I adored *bildungsromans*, books in which young protagonists came of age, or faced a challenge of self-sufficiency in order to grow. My copy of Cynthia Voigt's *Homecoming*, a story in which a young girl named Dicey is abandoned by her mother, with her three younger siblings, in a supermarket car park, was dog-eared from thumbing. Dicey sets out to travel on foot across America with her siblings and a map and seven dollars to find first their aunt and then, on discovering she has passed away, and that their mother is now in a mental institution, their long-lost grandmother. They forage in bins, and hunt and fish, and cross rivers and earn money washing windows, and eventually settle with their grandmother. Dicey's predicament and survival contained all my unbidden fantasies: a mother who becomes lost to her daughter, and a daughter who not only survives the abandonment but flourishes.

I wanted to leave my mother safely. To leave her and not put her in danger by my disappearance. The philosopher and psychoanalyst Luce Irigaray subverted the Freudian Oedipus theory so that the central battle in a woman's sexuality is not their struggle to overcome envy of the father's penis but a struggle to overcome the excess of their mother's love that they feel they have to bear. In Irigaray's myth the daughter yearns to leave, to follow her father, whom she sees exiting into the world as a separate being. But her battle is against the threat this poses to her mother: 'And the one doesn't stir without the other. When the one carries life, the other dies ... And what I wanted from you, Mother, was this: that in giving me life you still remain alive.'[17] Without assurance of my mother's happiness, I did not feel safe to leave her.

I felt as a child that my mother had not had a mother of her own to love her the way she needed to be loved. I wasn't sure why I felt this – her mother, Fay, had been present in our lives, an involved grandmother, until we emigrated – but it hovered in me, this sense of my mother freefalling, of her being outside the orbit of her family unit, not pulled in by the gravity of her parents' love.

Fay wasn't one of those grandmothers who cooked or helped in any seriously practical way, but she was there, good at storytelling and loving to Joni and me. When she did help, it often resulted in calamity. She drove down the wrong side of the road, taking us to ballet classes one day. She forgot to shut the car door on Joni's side another day, and it flew open dangerously as we rounded a corner. She couldn't fathom a remote control, work out a purse clasp. 'The hands don't clap sometimes,' my mother put it to me years later. My mother made up for the unpredictable incapacity of Fay by being overwhelmingly competent and capable. She emigrated across the world with two young children on her own, arriving at a city she did not know, sleeping on mattresses donated by a charity for new arrivals, finding houses for us to rent and schools for us to attend, going off to teach full-time at a university, and all while still grieving the end of her marriage.

Sometimes mothers manifested for her, to her great relief. When the arrival doors opened at Perth airport, she had expected to lug her suitcases and her two daughters on her own to the musty brown motor inn that was our home for the night in this unknown, scorching city, but there stood an older woman she had once met, the mother of a friend of Aaron's, who had gotten word that we were arriving. The woman was the opposite of Fay: independent, able to mobilise – an activist whose eldest son was in jail back in South Africa for his stand against Apartheid. She took Joni to May Day marches and invited us to her Communist

Party lunches. We called her our surrogate grandmother for those first few years.

Maxine had also found a mother back in South Africa whom she lost in the emigration, and that loss was a secondary injury. She still cries when she talks about this. Emily Nozipo Mtsolongo was, in the classifications of Apartheid South Africa, Maxine and Aaron's servant. She became their maid when they moved into their first apartment together after they married. They had not wanted a maid, partly because it seemed indulgent, being two healthy young people, and partly because they were liberal-thinking humanists and having a black maid was part and parcel of the Apartheid system. But Emily had been working for the previous tenants of their flat, and employing her would mean she could stay and continue to have a wage, which she asked of them. So they employed her, and my mother found in Emily a person who made her feel safe. Emily was an extremely large woman, with a mournful smile. She moved slowly on account of her size, which gave her a physical gentleness that matched her temperament.

She was from Soweto, in the townships where most of the black workers in Johannesburg came from. Her own children were back in those townships. Maxine loved Emily, and when she and Aaron were set to move to a house shortly before I was born she was devastated to find out that the strict Apartheid rules governing the movement of black citizens meant Emily could not move with them. 'I said to myself, *You will find Emily again*,' she told me years later. 'It was the only way I could leave her.'

Some time after I was born, before the divorce, my parents moved again, and my mother, probably sensing she would soon be a single mother, resolved to return to the flats and find Emily. But she was no longer working there. Maxine walked the streets of the suburb, asking the other women who worked as domestic servants if they knew her, and eventually she found her. This time they were not prepared to let each other go. She got a letter from her endocrinologist stating that Emily was the only person who knew how to assist her with her diabetic needs, and Emily was given the rubber stamp to move beyond where her pass allowed her, to the house where my mother and father would soon bury their marriage. Emily was a mother to me too, all the years after that until we left the country. I nestled high up on her bed, which had been raised on bricks to avoid the dark spirits of Zulu mythology, smelling the meaty, porridgey scent of the food she cooked in tin pots on her stove while Maxine was at work; I stood beside her, my hand enveloped in hers, for my first school photos. We all mourned leaving her. I mourned too, later as an adult, and felt deep guilt, for the knowledge that the mothering she did for us took her away from her own children. And I was filled with awe and gratitude at her capacity to have mothered so lovingly two white children whose culture directly oppressed her and her children. She died of a heart attack the year we arrived in Australia.

As for Fay, it was not that she was incapable of love. She loved Joni and me; I felt it. She found us hilarious; she hugged us close. I could not understand what had happened in her relationship with Maxine that meant my mother did not feel Fay's love, or that Fay did not give it.

I sensed my mother searching for a mother my whole life. She looked for them in the men she married – and in a sense found her own mother there, in that they left her freefalling too.

My mother often became lost to me. I don't mean she disappeared, or did not involve herself in my life: that she did with dedication. But her own sadness, the circumstance of my father leaving her and later my stepfather tormenting her, kept her often in a detached state of sorrow. Beneath her sharp humour ran a stream of distress that she failed to conceal.

The poet Adrienne Rich wrote of the complex feelings of self passed from mother to daughter: the 'cathexis between mother and daughter … is the great unwritten story'. Matrophobia, she said, is 'the fear of becoming one's mother'. It is the 'fear of conflicted identifications with and separation from the mother'. The mother must be, symbolically, severed in order for the daughter to survive: 'In a desperate attempt to know where mother ends and daughter begins, we perform radical surgery,' she wrote.[18] It was at last, in my move to Melbourne, with its brooding weather, laneways of grimy trellises, steam leaking from cafe grills and coffee roasters into snap-cold mornings, that I cut our cord. It wasn't the physical move that performed the radical surgery, though. It was in the way Melbourne led me to Gideon, and to becoming a mother myself. As in the myth of Demeter and Kore, I could not, with children and husband, be lured back from the underworld to assume a position of infancy by her side. I could only leave my world to visit her once in a while.

10

Being in the presence of a doctor never failed to elicit a kind of confessional weeping from me. Between choking sobs I described the past months of distress to the GP to whom I went for a formal referral to the psychiatrist whose name my father had given me.

'Do you have any support? A counsellor?' he asked.

I told him that I'd been in psychoanalysis for years.

'What do you mean by psychoanalysis – Freudian stuff?' He seemed taken aback, as though I had told him I was using a loom to weave my own undergarments. I was starting to feel confounded myself. I had been lying on Dr Parkes's couch for years, unravelling my memories and most fleeting and also persistent feelings, yet I was now in such a trough of despair that I was seeking medication, as I might if I had injured my body. Why had motherhood jolted me into now considering my distress not as a symptom of my personhood but as a corporeal injury? The doctor handed me some brochures on postnatal depression along with my referral, on which I saw he had scribbled the word *medication*.

Outside of the clinic, I took Reuben for a walk – autumn was setting in and the sky was sharp, cloudless. I stopped at a cafe for a takeaway coffee, and sat with him in a nearby park, his back warm against my body. While I was unsettled by the shift of perception that taking medication presented, in the act of getting the referral there was some mastery over the awful, relentless thrumming of my blood, the tightness of my throat.

It struck me: I was not, after all, helpless. I thought about how Dr Parkes never offered me a concrete course of action. He would never say, for example, *What about medication?* or *I suggest you get more sleep*, or *I think moving house would be a bad idea right now*. Many times during a session I had articulated a hope that a pill might make me better, and he had never answered with *Why don't you try?* I had taken his neutrality as tacit disapproval of chemical intervention.

As a foreign calm washed over me on that park bench, I realised his stance might be something else: a careful orchestration of enablement. I had brought to him over and over again my struggle with feeling unable to help myself, with feeling like a child in an adult world, lacking in agency, assertiveness, the ability to make things better for myself.

Instructing me to do something would be counter to the whole aim of our work together; his function was not to guide me or tell me the answer. Letting me discover my own authority and capacity for self-help had been his intention all along. The emergence of an intact self, replete with inner resources, is what psychoanalytic therapy aims for. 'A transformation which will lead gradually towards that birth which has at some point been postponed,' as the analyst and author Nini Herman wrote.[19] The postponed birth, she said, was the interruption to infant development that came about when a baby did not learn the difference between what was inside of them and outside of them; when they did not separate from their mother; and where that mother, the one who both frustrates and soothes, who evokes both hate and love, is in fact 'not so dismal an exchange for the cosy antechamber where everything ran nice and smoothly'.[20]

The GP seemed to consider my postnatal state a medical concern. Freud had rejected the idea of psychoanalysis as a means to address the medical: 'psychoanalysis is not a specialised branch of medicine,' he wrote in 1888 to Wilhelm Fleiss, '… we seek to enrich [the patient] from his own internal sources'.[21]

Dr Parkes had let me draw on my inner resources. Still, I felt angry with him. Or myself. I wasn't sure which. What if I had not been able to help myself? Would he have let me continue as I was?

I didn't care anymore for answers; it was time for some relief. I phoned and made an appointment with the psychiatrist.

On a Monday afternoon I left Reuben with Aaron, who was visiting. Leaving Reuben increased my anxiety threefold; a stream of rational thought – that he would be perfectly fine with my capable father who had a good stash of my breastmilk ready to warm up and mix in with porridge should Reuben get hungry – was swamped by a flood of irrational thought, encompassing everything from my father accidentally spilling all the milk to my father dropping dead while holding Reuben.

As though enacting my mental state, despite having been to the suburb of the psychiatrist countless times via what was essentially a straight main road, I became disoriented and turned down the wrong street a number of times. I became increasingly caught up on the matter of arriving precisely on time – both too late and too early seemed equally problematic – checking the car clock with obsessive attentiveness. Once I had parked and got out the car my anxiety transmuted into amnesia, and I was unable to remember the simple three-number lock code that the psychiatrist's receptionist had told me over the phone for entry into the terrace house. I had to phone my father and get him to riffle through the half-scrunched note papers in my study to find the scrap I'd jotted it down on.

By the time I perched myself tensely on the hard edge of the psychiatrist's otherwise cushioned settee, I was exhausted – it had been six months of operating in this state of permanent rigidity. I was brittle; fuelled by little more than adrenalin and the electric energy of panic. And so of course, in what was now becoming a familiar opening act, when the psychiatrist asked me to tell him about myself I cried. I could barely get a word out. I sobbed, and went through half a box of tissues, and tried to explain the past six months, and eventually settled into a shuddery kind of breathing and gave in to the softer middle of the chair.

'Why did you start seeing a psychoanalyst?' he asked me. The question took me by surprise somehow. In my present state of survival, I hadn't thought much about how I used to be, or what I used to feel, or even whether what was happening to me now was connected to anything that had happened to me before. But confronted with reflecting on what had taken me to the cream brick house in the leafy green suburb where Dr Parkes worked, I remembered that anxiety was not new to me. I remembered France, and high school, and the Buddhist therapist, and the increasing feelings of daily ennui, the bodily exhaustion, the nightmares, and then the trip to England with Gideon.

'It's likely, from the symptoms you describe,' said the psychiatrist, 'that you have what would be classified as peripartum depression. The *DSM* now recognises severe anxiety as part of that diagnosis. The cause is difficult to say, but I'd recommend a serotonin reuptake inhibitor, especially since you responded well to that in the past.'

The session was up. I left with a script for Zoloft, which I promptly filled at the nearest pharmacy before I could get firm cognisance over the idea of medicating myself again and perhaps start an argument with myself. I popped the first dose in the car, then phoned my father to find out if Reuben had survived my absence.

There was a week where I was wretched with head spins, insomnia. I yawned profusely, but they were strange, hollow yawns that left me feeling breathless. I discovered in a bout of googling that the head spins were called brain zaps, and were thought to be caused by alterations to neurotransmitters. What did this mean – that my mind-scaffolding was changing? I was overcome with bleakness; I felt detached from my body. I was tinged with the sense of helplessness that comes with thinking the thing that was supposed to make me better had made me worse. It was a dead-end kind of feeling, and, while I didn't have suicidal thoughts myself, I glimpsed momentarily a rational understanding of why someone might on this medication. But I had been warned by the psychiatrist that this may happen and to ride it out. All I needed to do was keep going and time would pass and it would work, I told myself. Reuben was growing and hungry, and days were a domino fall of breastfeeding, breakfast, breastfeeding, lunch, dinner, breastfeeding. The house smelled of cooked pear and warm Weet-Bix and boiled vegetables. I still had little appetite.

I had begun to think of my body as sick. I was sympathetic to myself and accepting of the slow passing of time and the idea of incremental improvement and cellular healing and respite as long as I thought of what I felt as bodily. My neurons adjusting, getting used to the inhibition of the reuptake of my serotonin, which was a concept I found both abstract and inconceivable in its almost double negativity: Was serotonin good or bad? Was it that I needed more or less? Why was it being uptaken in the first place and where to?

Months later, I investigated the *DSM*, which the psychiatrist had mentioned: the *Diagnostic and Statistical Manual of Mental Disorders*. It was updated every few decades, and in its latest version two significant things had been added to how it framed the kind of experience I had had.

While there was no stand-alone classification for postnatal anxiety, symptoms of anxiety and panic had now been recognised as being part of a 'postpartum onset major depressive episode'. The timeframe for diagnosis had also been extended: symptoms might show up *during* pregnancy: 'Fifty percent of "postpartum" major depressive episodes actually begin prior to delivery. Thus, these episodes are referred to collectively as peripartum episodes. Women with peripartum major depressive episodes often have severe anxiety and even panic attacks.'[22]

When I looked further into the history of the *DSM*'s broader changes I discovered the archaeological remains of an intellectual battle much like the one I was having with myself about what had happened to me. The *DSM* had been created in 1952 in America to give doctors and psychiatrists a standardised classification scheme for mental illness: clusters of symptoms gathered into categories. Before this, from as far back as the nineteenth century, American doctors dealing with mental illness worked mainly in asylums with patients who had severe mental dysfunctions, and these were understood somatically; as the result of physical impairment or disease. Injury to the organ of the brain was considered the source of behavioural symptoms. Those doctors relied on a diagnostic list of only twenty-two classifications.

The *DSM* came about as psychiatry broadened its reach beyond mental asylums and into 'normal' life, with a growing recognition that it didn't just take a blow to the head or a brain infection to cause mental maladjustment. Post World War Two, servicemen, including psychiatrists who had served, were showing a range of emotional problems that indicated environmental stress also had a significant impact on a person. These servicemen were functional but disturbed. Institutionalisation was not an optimal setting for their recovery.

Instead, many began treatment with a psychoanalytic approach. Freud had gained a foothold in Europe earlier in the century, and his ideas had spread to America. The psychiatrist Adolf Meyer, for whom 'mental illness' was the reaction of a personality to psychological, social and biological factors, had been especially influential. Psychoanalytic therapy offered a treatment that addressed these men's injured minds rather than their brains; it could be done within a community setting, and it was showing good recovery rates.[23]

As psychiatry itself expanded its influence postwar (with recognition of the significance of emotional trauma came improved status and rank for psychiatrists in military services, and men who might have gone into other medical specialties were now interested in the field) so did a realisation that there was a spectrum of mental health suffering, and that some of the general population who were not at the extreme end could benefit from talking therapy. By 1946, the American Board of Psychiatry had formalised psychoanalytic theory as the leading school of thought in mental health treatment.[24]

War, humanity's most brutal invention, can be blamed then for psychoanalysis blooming, for galvanising the diagnoses of mental illness in a Freudian language of neuroses, resistances and underlying conflicts. (It also explains why it had taken until 1994, with the publication of *DSM-IV*, for any kind of perinatal language to enter the manual. That version had added the words 'postpartum onset' to the classification of a major depressive episode. As a manual initially designed to assess soldiers going into service, and then to assess the symptoms frequently being presented by World War Two active-duty servicemen and veterans, its incarnation was inherently masculine.)

The five versions of the *DSM* that took shape over the next sixty-one years saw the Freudian presence eroded, as tension developed between a psychological and a bio-medical approach to mental experience in psychiatry. By the 1960s psychoanalysis was losing supporters, its research and resource funding diminishing under a perception that its studies lacked rigour. In the *DSM-II*, in 1968, the psychoanalytic influence on diagnoses was watered down: the focus returned to symptoms rather than their underlying *conflicts*.

In the lead-up to the *DSM-III* in 1980, the stage was set for its psychoanalytic purge. Freud's concept of the ways an individual's past, their unconscious thinking, could impact on their behaviour was too unspecific, too subjective for a field that was looking to diagnose categorically. The purpose of the *DSM*, after all, had been to arrive at some kind of uniformity among diagnosticians, in a field extending its reach into the psychopathology of everyday life.

And there came a scandal: the Rosenhan experiment, in which a number of 'pseudo-patients' got themselves admitted to psychiatric institutions with schizophrenia diagnoses by feigning hallucinations. The definitional terms of psychiatry were unclear, came the criticism. How could we tell the difference between sane and insane? Science-minded psychiatrist Robert Spitzer was put at the helm of a revised *DSM*, whose board was still largely composed of psychoanalysts. Spitzer explained his stance to the *New Yorker* magazine in 2005: 'Rather than just appealing to authority, the authority of Freud, the appeal was: Are there studies? What evidence is there?'

Spitzer faced a tough crowd in trying to convince the Freud-friendly board to pass the revisions, but they were approved, and *DSM-III* moved even more distinctly away from cause and toward symptoms, with a tick-box model that would assure agreement of diagnoses between psychiatrists. Whether or not the diagnoses represented real diseases or conditions, or only amounted to meaningless labels for connected symptoms became, and remains, the biggest criticism of the *DSM*.

Once you start reducing anything to aggregates, to median scores, to words that attain the greatest breadth of mutual recognition, you lose the nuances that make those things different. Amber becomes orange becomes off-white becomes yellow. It all becomes yellow in the end.

When *DSM-5* came out, in 2013, Dr Steven Hyman, former director of the American National Institute of Mental Health (NIMH) commented: 'We have to understand the *DSM* as a set of guidelines to diagnosis of often very serious disorders, but not as the bible of psychiatry ... the brain is the most complicated organ in the history of human scientific endeavor. And we need to be able to approach it with an open mind.'[25]

His successor, Dr Thomas R Insel, was more emphatic, critical not only of the impossibility of reducing complex human symptomatology to neat descriptors but of the science behind the *DSM*: 'People think that everything has to match *DSM* criteria, but you know what? Biology never read that book.'[26]

But Hyman, Insel and their NIMH colleagues, although looking to change the status quo, were hardly after a return to Freud. Insel's focus, after taking on the directorship, was to bring scientific validity to psychiatric diagnostics. He wanted to return to causes and move away from symptoms, and to do so with a focus on the biological bases of behaviour. He headed up a research framework called Research Domain Criteria (RDoC), which studies mental-disorder constructs through genes, molecules, cells, brain circuits, physiology and behaviour. Research done under the RDoC framework looks to diagnose people according to categories such as cognitive function (what are a person's visual and auditory perceptions like, for example) and social process functions (what are their responses in interpersonal settings) rather than giving them *DSM* diagnoses, which they believe are less useful in their homogeneity.

Clinical researchers, who use *DSM-5* as their framework, haven't been pleased with this new approach. According to an analysis in 2017 by *Nature* magazine, the number of clinical trials funded by the NIMH has fallen by 45 per cent since the agency began to focus on the biological roots of disease rather than on the broader symptoms set out by the *DSM*.[27] It is as though to study the human mind as simultaneously biological, mental and behavioural poses an impossibility.

Being able to classify a person's mental experience has some practical justifications for medical insurance, for psychiatric research developments and funding, and for determining outcomes in court cases. In Australia, it is used alongside the World Health Organization's *International Classification of Diseases: classification of mental and behavioural disorders, 10th revision*

(ICD-10) – a guide that took over in 1949, not long after the establishment of the WHO, from previous statistical attempts to draw together uniform classifications for causes of death in a global common language, and that provides the relevant codes for health insurance use. Many practitioners use both: some feel the *ICD* allows more clinical discretion in diagnosing, and some feel the *DSM* offers better research classifications.[28] Increasingly, the *ICD* is considered a more reliable resource, free from the institutional forces that imbue the *DSM*, created, as it is, by the American Psychiatric Association.

When I'd gone to a GP to get a referral for Dr Parkes all those years ago, I hadn't yet identified what I was experiencing as anxiety. The GP had asked me: 'Why do you need to see a therapist?' I had struggled to answer him. I'd said something like, 'Life stuff.' He had looked at me over the top of his bifocals, and I'd understood he needed outward expressions of my suffering or he could not assign a health insurance item to my referral. 'Insomnia,' I said. 'I am not sleeping. Or eating.'

That was all true, but those physical symptoms were the least of my problems. Nowhere in his manual did it list the grief of fathers leaving, or the impossibility of going as far into the adult world as France because you could not be at a distance from your mother.

A diagnosis brought nothing to my work with Dr Parkes. He viewed my experience as part of the continuum of my life; as an extension of the feelings I'd had before becoming a mother and would now have as a mother, and our work together continued on that basis. But it offered me a language to talk about how bad things had been.

I told some friends that I had postnatal anxiety. Perinatal depression, as the *DSM* would have it, didn't seem to capture the experience for me, putting the emphasis on feelings of lowness, which I did of course have, above the incapacitating panic. One friend, Anna, whom I confided in, was pregnant with her first baby. She organised for me to have coffee with another friend of hers who had been hospitalised for her perinatal depression. The three of us met at a cafe and swapped stories; Anna a sort of Oprah between us, facilitating our confessions of madness and recovery. In a few months, Anna was less facilitator than fellow panel guest. She gave birth, and a mania of anxiety set in. She jumped on the trampoline at night to stop her thoughts. She went onto medication too. After that she would visit me from time to time to bathe with her baby. They had no bath at their house and she found lying with the baby in water calmed her. Anna spoke about her anxiety in chemical terms: it was set off by hormonal changes; the doctors had put her on antidepressants and anxiolytics.

Meanwhile, after about a week, the head spins and insomnia subsided, and it wasn't that I felt euphoric but there was no panic. My bodily exhaustion lifted. Even if I woke to feed Reuben five times in a night, I felt functional and alert in the morning. My jaw relaxed; I hadn't realised how tightly I had been clenching it but now when I chewed, the tenderness I had been feeling along my jawbone had gone. I got hungry. I watched television and cooked, and a few months later I read a magazine, and then I read a book. I went to Dr Parkes and I didn't cry. But I wasn't sure this was a good thing.

11

Two years later, Gideon and I decided we wanted a second child. Difficult as my postnatal experience had been, I wanted to give Reuben a sibling – I couldn't imagine my childhood without the company of Joni. And the love I felt for Reuben, the yearning for his little body, his duck-soft hair and dimpled legs, the pleasure of watching his mind grow: I wanted more of that. But I could not deny that a repeat of the anxiety I'd had with Reuben would break me, especially with two children to care for.

I had taken myself off medication a few months before I fell pregnant, sure that the panic had passed. I seemed stable. I had read that up to 40 per cent of women who experience postnatal depression with the birth of one child will experience it with another.[29] Still, I bargained with myself, perhaps the awful tangle I had gotten myself into after Reuben was first-time motherhood. The power of cognitive dissonance.

Gideon, with his characteristic nonchalant disposition, brushed off my concerns about it happening again. 'Look! Everything is fine now. Whatever happens, we'll get through it,' he said. Perhaps I had been too competent, I considered. It had felt, that first year, that nothing was holding up, but we were once again going through the motions of living: by the end of that year we were going out for dinner with friends again, the house was always in order, the dog walked. I had even begun working again.

The second time around, there would be no dithering about sleep schedules, I told myself, as if this had been the real problem.

And if all failed, I would go back onto medication if I began to feel bad. And as soon as I had resolved my worry on this point, I fell pregnant again.

Like clockwork, the nausea took hold of me for seven weeks, followed by the same pelvic ligament condition that had afflicted me with Reuben. With Reuben to look after, I couldn't spend this pregnancy lying down, but the pain was insurmountable. I felt myself curl into my own mind again, the experience of time passing excruciatingly slowly as I focused more on my every feeling than on life as it happened. I managed to get us into the car to drop Reuben at day care, but once again I could not do the shopping, cooking, cleaning and domestic ordering that would have given me a sense of command over the chaos of daily life. I worked for myself now, but even in the comfort of my own home I couldn't sit at my desk editing books for hours on end; and I couldn't, once again, get the baby's room ready myself, which felt in itself like an anxiety dream. Gideon bathed Reuben at night, carried him into his room and sat him on my lap so I could dry him and be part of his bedtime routine. If he called out at night Gideon went to him. Often I cried in the dark of our bedroom when Gideon went. 'Mummy's here,' I'd say into the monitor, feeling the distance between us as a valley I couldn't cross.

On the days when I had Reuben with me, we read together on the couch, or I set him up with Play-Doh or paint at a little table I placed beside an armchair that I was relatively comfortable in. I took him to art classes, and winced with pain sitting on the hard bench doing papier-mache with him, and limped around play centres, perching on mini-slides and leaning on cubby houses. At night I collapsed into bed with relief, and lay on my side with icepacks strung along my lower back, a deep ache setting in to my hips. I longed for codeine.

This time, at least, I had more control over the birth experience. I had gotten private health cover for obstetrics. I opted to have Noah by caesarean, backed by the reasoning that, statistically, second babies are heavier. I didn't feel I could go through a traumatic labour like I had had with Reuben again. In any case, I couldn't stand. It was never going to be an active labour.

As the date approached for Noah's birth, I felt my mood lower. I put it down to my incapacitation: it had been months since I had been to the cinema, or taken a walk, or cooked. We were living on frozen lasagnes. Still, I was crying a lot again. No panic, but enough crying to be worrying. I cried when I said goodbye to Reuben at day care; I cried when I kissed him goodnight. I cried when I folded the clothes that had been his and would be Noah's. On Dr Parkes's couch, I talked about how awful I felt for Reuben that I was unable to do things with him anymore. How I felt I was abandoning him. My idea of a sibling being a gift for him had somehow transformed into being an attack on him.

'A mother can't have more than one baby in your world,' Dr Parkes said, and I saw that I feared Reuben would experience the baby's arrival as a replacement of him. That he would think me dead, gone to him, when I attended to the baby. In my world, the world in which my father had left us for someone else, there wasn't room for new loves. One love catastrophically destroyed the other. And one baby forced to grow up by the arrival of another baby was severed from the mother eternally. My separation fantasies permeated my thinking, set the direction of my inner compass. Dr Parkes gave me rational explanations for feelings in me that felt irrational. When I understood the story behind these overpowering feelings, they faded.

The obstetrician, on the other hand, felt my state was physiological. 'Your oestrogen will drop after the baby is born. Lowered oestrogen is a clear trigger for anxiety. We know, in your case, this is what has happened. The likelihood of it happening again is high. I think you ought to seriously consider going onto antidepressants now, just a low dose.'

I could see the fuzzy outline of Noah on a monitor when he was saying this. It was impossible not to imagine he was Reuben.

It was necessary for him to be Reuben or else I would be replacing Reuben with someone else. I understood this thought running through my mind as the obstetrician spoke, and I wanted to protest: *No, you don't understand. The anxiety isn't chemical; it's me.*

Noah was born, raised from my numbed abdomen, in under an hour. We had sat around a waiting room with people going for day surgery – wisdom teeth removal and cataract ops – and then been called into a small cubicle, where we went through pre-operative checks and changed: me into a hospital gown, Gideon into scrubs. Clinical precision and procedure had replaced the primitive energy of my labour, but the order and predictability of events was far preferable for me than the prolonged uncertainty and agony of Reuben's birth. I held Noah and put him to my breast and cried from overwhelming love for my new son. He looked nothing like Reuben and everything like a unique, different person: smaller, less hair and tinier features.

That evening, Gideon brought Reuben to meet his baby brother. I was high, morphine coursing through me. My two perfect sons – Reuben was intact; I had not destroyed him. And he seemed to look at his baby brother with affection and interest. I watched as he stood by Noah's plastic crib and pressed his favourite sleep toy, a yellow giraffe blankie, against the side for Noah to see. It seemed possible I might be all right; that all the talking I had done on the couch had helped me understand my previous anxiety enough to keep it away this time. This time I would be able to lift my baby; this time I would eat and stay strong.

All the differences between my birth experience with Reuben and with Noah represented proof to me that this time I would not succumb, I would not disintegrate. I had a huge room, light and airy and with a comfortable queen-sized bed and my own private bathroom. I had been in a public hospital with Reuben – entirely adequate but with the expected gruel-ish dinner slop on fraying plastic-ware, jaundiced light; displeasures that I had been numb to in any case, felled as I was by my sorrow and panic. This time,

I was highly attuned to sensory pleasure. I felt hungry – the food was veritably gourmet: perfectly cooked tender steaks served on ceramic plates with sides of fresh green asparagus, peas. I held Noah to my breast, the two of us falling easily into breastfeeding, while I ate my steak and chatted to friends on the phone. I could pick Noah up, and move around; I was not helpless with pain as I had been after Reuben's birth. On my final night in hospital, as was offered for private patients, we were sent to stay at a five-star hotel, and Reuben and Gideon came too. Gideon took Reuben swimming in the hotel pool, and we dined on meals covered by silver cloches and sunk together as a family of four onto well-starched sheets and goose-down duvets. Before I went to sleep that night I turned to Gideon and said: 'This time is different.'

And it was, in that this time it was not the postbox but my hospital bag. I looked at it and could not make sense of where its contents should go. Washing. The nightgowns were for the washing, still smelling faintly of hospital air. I saw a pile of clothes on our bedroom floor, and another pile on the bathroom floor, and I walked into the laundry and found six piles in there. I walked back to our bedroom. I was still holding the nightgown. I walked back to the laundry. I stood in the laundry. I thought, *Washing. When will I do the washing?* and the thought was somehow catastrophic, sent a shot of terror through me. With each thought came piles of thoughts, a to-do list I couldn't quiet. Change nappy, feed, eat, shower, sleep, washing, dinner, Reuben. Where was Reuben? I wanted to get into bed with Reuben and hold him. *He mustn't think I won't hold him anymore.* 'Hello, my baby sweetheart,' I said to him. I felt an awful dread settle on me – how would I hold two children?

In the shower I stood and let the water run over my face and thought about getting out of the shower and a new list began: take Panadol – *It is important to keep your pain in check*, the nurse had said; drink water – *It is important to stay hydrated*, the doctor had said. My milk was coming in – I had rock-hard breasts: *Put icepacks on to reduce the engorgement*, the midwife had said, *and then heat packs when feeding to help the milk let down.* When had Noah's nappy been changed? *Keep him very dry*, the doctor had said, seeing the start of a painful nappy rash. *Watch for crampy feelings in your legs*, the obstetrician had said. *Deep-vein thrombosis is a risk after a caesar.*

A maternal and child health nurse visited me at home for a check-up. She was not reassuring and kind like my nurse with Reuben had been. The crying had begun again for me, and I cried while she checked Noah's remaining umbilical cord. 'Your generation think too much about things,' she said.

At the hospital Noah had slept all day and at night in chunks of hours, but since the first night home he had opened his eyes at 7 pm and begun to scream. I put him on my breast. He stopped screaming. I kept him there for thirty minutes and took him off again. He screamed. I put him back on. Peace. I took him off again. He screamed. We gave him a dummy. He still screamed. Gideon put Reuben to bed and I made sure I was in the room to see him off to sleep as I had always been, but now with Noah attached to me, still sucking but at least quiet. I returned to my room and took him off. He screamed. I lay in the bed with him and let him breastfeed there beside me, fighting my closing eyes, desperate to sleep. Rules ran though my head. *Sharing a sleep surface with a baby can increase the risk of Sudden Infant Death.* I told myself to stay awake. Gideon lay beside us and dozed. I tried taking Noah off again. He screamed.

At 3 am, I thought of a person on a cliff clinging on with one hand waiting for a rescue team. I remembered a friend saying her baby would only settle in his car capsule. I sent Gideon to the car to bring in the capsule. I got forty blissful minutes of half-sleep, one hand rocking Noah in the car capsule that Gideon had set up between us in the bed. Then Noah began screaming again. I looked around the room, startled. Was it Reuben? No, I had a baby again, I remembered. Maybe Noah was starving; maybe I wasn't producing enough milk yet. I sent Gideon to the kitchen to make up a bottle of formula. We had never used formula. *Breastfeeding works on supply and demand. Using formula will prevent you building up your milk supply*, the books had said. But I thought I would die from exhaustion. Better an interrupted milk supply than a dead mother, I thought. Noah drank half the bottle Gideon offered him and, in the quiet, a new list began in my head: sterilise bottles, pump breasts to keep up supply, do washing, drink water. Then he started screaming again. The sun began to rise, Reuben woke and came to our room, and Noah fell into a deep, quiet sleep, so peaceful and so silent that it gave me at last the space to drift in and out of the kind of half-thought that allows panic to bloom fully and rapaciously.

'I am not well,' I told the obstetrician over the phone in a thin voice.

'How bad is it?' he asked.

'I can't eat. I can't stop crying,' I managed to get out.

'I would like you to consider going in to hospital for care,' said the obstetrician.

Gideon was clanging about in the background, hauling out the KitchenAid from under the sink. His way of mobilising was to bake.

I told the obstetrician I would think about it, but I knew I wouldn't. I was whirring on an electric treadmill of thought that told me I couldn't leave Reuben because I had abandoned Reuben by having another baby.

I phoned Dr Parkes. 'I am not well,' I told him. 'I can't eat. I can't stop crying. The obstetrician wants me to go to a mother–baby unit, but I can't leave Reuben. This is worse than the first time. Now I am trapped,' I told him.

'Would you like to come and see me?' he asked.

'I am putting myself back on medication,' I told him.

'Would you like to come and see me?' he asked again.

'Fine. I'll come and see you. But I'm putting myself back on medication.' It had been a year of no medication, and I had been okay, but clearly I wasn't now. I thought back to pregnancy with Noah. I hadn't felt wonderful. But that was pregnancy, wasn't it? I had been immobile again with the pelvis thing: who would be on top of the world with that? I had cried a lot at small things. The man at the supermarket who accused me of taking his lettuce. The woman who gave me the finger in the car park. Who wouldn't cry?

In the bathroom where a new pile of washing now sat on the floor I found the script I had kept in case of exactly this situation. *Break in case of emergency.*

I breastfed Noah on the couch while Gideon's bread rose in the oven. Reuben cuddled in beside us, and I managed with my free arm to hold up a book, which I read to him. Out loud I read the story but in my head I said over and over again, *It will be better soon, it will be better soon.*

We all piled into the car and went to the shops, where Gideon went off with Reuben to buy milk while I sat sobbing on a bench outside the chemist with Noah in the car capsule beside me and waited for the script to be filled.

Released again by a pill. All those increments of hours in which Dr Parkes had closely observed the things I expressed in my relationship with him: my words, gestures, dreams. All his hypotheses about what lay under guard in me, in the hope that bringing it to light would loosen its convoluted grip, and here I was again, saved by chemical intervention.

PART 2

12

In another sense, here is where this story started: a year or so after that moment waiting on the bench with my second baby for my second round of medication. With Joni, in a cafe near where she worked, this time. In a suburb in Melbourne that had been overlaid so many times with different identities that its urban decay, its warehouse steel, its rock band posters and *For Sale* signs, its glossy, glassed privatised hospitals now coexisted in a kind of messy collage around us. Place is always important to this story; everything I say is important to what I mean, in the end, if I'm going to consider this all psychoanalytically. We were about to order coffee when this woman leaned over and intercepted the waiter.

'Have you seen a neurologist yet?' she asked him.

I couldn't help listening in, not least because they were conversing over my head.

His answer sounded flippant, the tenor of a man not wanting to seem grave: 'I'm on the wait-list. You know brain doctors: tumours, strokes … the dying people get to go first. Mine's not urgent.'

Joni was a clinical researcher at a hospital, and all around us were people potentially unwell, recovering, dying, visiting the dying. The overflow from the hospital cafeteria. I wondered if anyone near us was one of the *inconsiderates* taking up the neurologist's wait-list. Also, what could be *not-urgent* that involved a brain? Brains. They'd been on my mind for a while; surely that was an old neurologists' joke.

We ordered, and I watched the waiter walk away, wondered how he could go about his daily business with a *brain thing* on hold. I would have been knocking down the doctor's door for an MRI. But I'm certain of imminent demise within my body at any moment. It's always seemed to me that bodies are predisposed to collapse. I avoid knowing too much about the corporeal: each time I've accrued any working sense of an organ – say, the pancreas, during Maxine's explanation of her diabetes when I was a child – it has seemed to me to be sheer dumb luck that any of us survive at all. The body is a more complex version of that game Mouse Trap: a Rube Goldberg contraption holding up survival via a delicate balance of loops, pathways, connections and vessels.

Only the day before I had read about a young journalist who overnight had become strangely unwell because of one small glitch in the way her body responded to a virus. 'It was like she had a psychotic disorder,' I told Joni. The journalist had had paranoid thoughts, delusions – the first doctor she saw diagnosed her as bipolar and put her on antipsychotics.

I could see my sister processing my words: her great, ever-questioning mind filtering the information like a sand sifter. I ploughed on.

'Then she saw a doctor who tried that cognitive screening test on her – you know, the one they give Alzheimer's patients, where they get you to draw a clock? She put all the numbers squished up on the right-hand side, as though the left didn't exist, which meant it was neurological not psychiatric.'

'So what was it?' Joni asked. She's never one to let a story go by on generalisations. Specifics are the key to truth, as far as she's concerned. Scientific inquiry, the rigour of evidence. Don't go telling her you swear by reiki.

'Auto-immune something or other. To do with the something, something receptor?' The register of my voice was going up idiotically. 'A disease that was causing her brain to attack itself.'

I received slow, patient blinks.

'The bit I'm interested in was this: she said her care was more sympathetic when they decided it was neurological. They were nicer to her because her brain was sick, not her mind. As if the mind and brain are separate.'

'Course they're not,' she said, buttering her newly delivered toast.

'Aha!' I snapped, too loudly. 'You think they are connected!' I was aware that I was being unnecessarily accusatory; the mouse trap had come down.

But she went on, reasonably. 'You've got to be careful not to talk about the mind and the body as though they are innately able to control each other. You know – *think positive and you'll get better* – that kind of thing.'

I looked out the bay window at the people pushing against the hot summer wind to get back to their refrigerated offices and felt a twinge of envy at their singular routine. I would rush back soon to Noah, who was with Aaron between patients. I still felt a phantom leak of milk from my breasts, the tingle of a letdown, thinking of him, even though he had weaned himself a few months earlier. We drank our coffees in silence.

Joni was passionate about exposing 'woo', as it is known among those with a vigilance for scientific methodology. The stuff that charlatans make a buck from – unfounded therapies with no evidential basis: detoxes and vitamin C injections, crystals. As a nurse, she'd seen too many cancer patients in her care lose money, gain false hope, approach death remaining in painful denial of their mortality, sometimes die needlessly, the opportunity for medical intervention shunned for a 'natural' alternative with no real efficacy.

I lacked Joni's vast body of biological knowledge and her science education, having majored in English, studied Law. At school I'd avoided biology at all costs, fell into a stupor of boredom in physics classes. I fainted during the diabetes test when I was pregnant with Reuben merely because I was thinking about the fact that I have blood.

But I was no health hippie. Hospitals made me feel safe. It was my very inability to dwell on my innards – and the conviction that medical professionals base their practices on things that have occurred with other people's innards – that made me trust the medical fraternity absolutely. When I'd had both Reuben and Noah, I'd felt more at ease with the smell of antiseptic and the cold assurance of an electric monitor-beep than I would have among the familiarity of my house, with the dog poking its head in and the ordinary chaos of my kitchen at hand. I would volunteer to be placed on a gurney and operated on any day rather than trying a herb or a prayer. The providence of being alive was fortune enough – I wanted to be near the people with the tools and the knowledge to hold me together should one of my screws come loose.

And yet I had been thinking lately how for nearly a quarter of my life I had given myself over to psychoanalysis, to understanding my mind on the couch of Dr Parkes, an act so personal and subjective and bound to language that it seemed to exist in a different galaxy to the certainty and measurability of medicine and science.

I thought about my unseeable mind and how the whole process of its demise after my sons were born was connected with my body: giving birth. And how my body in the past four years had so clearly evidenced my mind-crumble: the back pain from holding my self tensely all the time; my unexpectedly concave post-baby stomach from never having an appetite. And how at the worst of both crises I had taken drugs to feel better.

They had seemed to have no clear cause, no neatly divisible borders, those postnatal crises. Complex vines of why and how I was still trying to disentangle: sleep deprivation, hormones, genetics, memories of my own babyhood when Aaron left, fragments of Maxine's grief trickled down to me.

I thought about how I – how could I put it? – I had reached for metaphor so often to articulate what it had felt like. Metaphor is the Latin *meta* (over, across, beyond) and *phor* (to carry). It carries a new, unknown experience into an old word. It was falling, falling, falling into a well of helplessness; it was not finding anything to cling onto on my way down, not Gideon, or my writing, or even my overwhelming love for Reuben and Noah.

Was there a part of the organ of my brain that had been affected at a cellular level by the bodily experience of motherhood? I had become quite literal about the whole thing, imagining a pin-drop on my brain, a flag; something that could be excised. The language of postnatal depression was corporeal: it is an *illness*, a *condition*. Was it simply a failing of my body?

Or had it happened, as I had wagered all those hours on the couch, because of my emotional make-up? My history and early-life experience? The part of me that, going on Freud and those who came after him, was formed of pre-rational thoughts in early infancy, and that held reeling unconscious desires and instincts and that would only truly release me from their convoluted ways if I could riddle them out through the talking cure?

'I'm starting to understand what happened to me postnatally,' I told Joni. 'I think going to Dr Parkes has helped me see the emotional origins of some of it.'

'Yeah? That's great,' she responded, but something was off. I always knew when Joni wasn't being honest; she'd get this funny look, her mouth sort of freezing.

'What's the matter?' I asked her.

She was hesitant; I could see she was trying not to offend me, but that she also wanted to wield her knowledge like a sharp, clean knife. 'Have you heard of confirmation bias?' she asked. I nodded but she went ahead and explained it to me anyway. 'It's a well-known cognitive phenomenon. It's when you select and interpret information in a way that confirms what you want to believe.'

'But you agree that psychoanalysis works? I mean, it can work for some people?' In my voice I registered the tenor of begging.

What was it in me that so feared her saying no? It wasn't just that I wanted to be right, or to have my years on the couch validated. There was something more at stake here, and it was existential. I did not believe in God. Psychoanalysis had offered me the promise of meaning. If we were only our bodies and the evolutionary tics of our forebears, if we were only the luck of DNA, of learned behaviour, if only survival was at stake, I could not bear it. Like writing and reading, the experience of psychoanalysis gave me the opportunity to live and one day die with a sense of having come to know something of myself. I couldn't shut the door on my postnatal experience and put it down to no more than my body being flooded with hormones. Or was it that I feared her scepticism because I knew that in the worst of my anxiety I had hated Dr Parkes for failing me? I had needed immediate relief. Lying on the couch hadn't cut it.

I was nervous, tapping my teaspoon wildly against my coffee cup. Joni always bore the power to dash my sense of reality with evidence studiously gathered from her vast home library or network of highly qualified scientist friends. I was more prone to trying and failing to remember a line from a poem to argue a point and then calling her at 2 am with my *esprit d'escalier.*

'It has no scientific basis,' she said, calmly and directly.

13

What if Joni was right, and Freud's concept of an unconscious mind that must be made conscious to release us from its tyranny had no truth to it at all? If it wasn't scientific, could it still be true? Had I been duped by its intellectualism, its associations with literature and language and poetry, into believing it could help me understand that which was simply and purely biological: genetics, hormones, neurochemistry? Or was it just that I had not yet drawn out far enough the threads of story from my life, my family? Had I not gone far enough yet?

'All sciences are based on observation and experience that are mediated by our psychical apparatus. However, as our science takes this apparatus itself as an object, the analogy ends here.'[30]

I thought about Freud's words, scribbled into my notebook, sitting amid the detritus of my bedroom floor, where dust balls gathered over the week were now scattering violently from the impact of several small Marvel Comic figurines that Noah was tossing about in play. I fancied it would make a good slow-motion video, the rise and fall of those particles in the buttery lamp light.

Years before Reuben was born, I had read about the psychoanalyst Marion Milner, who had become best known for her ideas about the value of becoming attuned to our unconscious thoughts and feelings through a method of introspective journaling. Milner, who wrote under the name Joanna Field, felt that people who had needed to protect themselves emotionally from more primitive states of thinking – states in which their sense of boundaries, between themselves and others, and also in their environments, are diminished – might become cut off from their more imaginative, unconscious selves, and out of touch with their self-deceptions. A child, for example, whose mother is emotionally ill, might so strongly assert their logical, cognitive thinking to preserve a sense of difference between themselves and their frightening mother. But this self-preservation, Milner said, sacrificed their imaginative self; the self that emerged in dreams and in fleeting thoughts that would give way to true understanding of one's personal sense of meaning. She advocated keeping diaries of stream-of-consciousness thoughts, a focus on becoming attuned to the minutiae of your own mind's experiences.

Milner's brother, Patrick Blackett, was a physicist working in experimental particle physics. He won the Nobel Prize for Physics for his investigations of cosmic rays, using a cloud chamber – a particle detector used to pick up ionising radiation. Blackett had invented a way of getting the chamber to compress more rapidly, making it even more sensitive.

Two siblings, each interested in matter indecipherably small, but Blackett's was a material interest, while Milner's required observing the psychic apparatus itself – the mind – and that came with the inherent subjectivity that would foil any scientific endeavour. Milner herself had lamented:

> I had become disgusted with science for giving me what was not in its power to give. One warm summer evening, steaming out of London on a week-end train, I caught a glimpse through the window of a fat old woman in apron and rolled sleeves surveying her grimy back garden from the door-step. At once I was seized with an impulse to know more about her, and then began wondering what the scientists who deal with different phases of social life could tell me. I had even got as far as resolving to read some books on sociology, when it suddenly dawned on me that

> that was not at all what I wanted: I wanted to know that woman as a person, a unique individual, not as a specimen.[31]

I watched Noah. What thing done or not done, I wondered, in the maddened way that I had wondered at so many inexplicable events since having children, had caused his current sleeplessness? Had he napped too much in the day? Had I given him caffeine inadvertently? Let him watch too many screens? His brother was fast asleep. I drew up mentally a comparative itemisation of foods consumed and activities taken by each of them, hoping to hit upon an obvious standard deviation.

Perhaps it was also a kind of madness of motherhood that had entered me and caused me to listen to Joni's scepticism. Motherhood had driven me to feel more acutely than ever before a need for unequivocal answers. It was a state in which science, with its reverence for measurability, its attention to the removal and addition of factors, its scalpel-grade accuracy, had appealed to me more than ever, and yet it was a state in which hardly any experiences could be held to scientific measure. Parenting was mired in a glut of un-researched conjecture about sleep and feeding behaviour, and it had driven me batty with its looping strands of ad hoc advice. Never before had I been plunged into a wilder wood of anecdote than in my desperate attempts to get sleep in those early months with Reuben. I had googled questions that I was embarrassed to admit. *Will my baby settle better when he can roll? Will my baby cry less when the car seat faces forward?* I thought with shame how I had at times regarded my children like machines; hoped beyond hope that there was a simple, equation-based solution to any challenge, to any quirk of their personhood or body. It was easy to see how Joni's commitment to scientifically validated information brought its own kind of peace. Clear causation. Joni didn't have children; she hadn't needed motherhood to push her to wanting evidence of what worked and what didn't.

Oh, but for the state of not-knowing that the poet Keats had famously called negative capability, in which one could give in to feelings of uncertainty rather than reach for fact or solution. Keats believed this state to be optimal for creating art. My father, going on his intellectual muse Wilfred Bion, believed this state optimal for good psychoanalytic work: tolerate pain and upheaval in order to grow. I had no doubt that surrendering to a state of not-knowing would give way to more relaxed parenting. But where did it fit into an urgent inquiry into my self? Was it reasonable to expect me to endure the depth of panic I had felt after both children were born in order to understand it? Was that what psychoanalytic work expected of me? Was I a psychoanalytic failure because I had gone the clear-cut chemical route?

I camped us both out in bed and put the television on, settling on the most neutral program I could find at that dark hour of adult programming: the home-shopping channel. Noah was quickly entranced by a demonstration of a miracle pot cleaner.

The myth of Freud is pervasive. He was a lecherous, sex-obsessed charlatan. He was a self-experimenting quack. Rarely is he remembered as a staunchly materialist scientist who looked to biology for his study of the mind, and who conceded that the times were against him in that field: 'we cannot guess what answers it will return in a few dozen years to the questions we have put to it. They may be of a kind which will blow away the whole of our artificial structure of hypotheses,' he wrote in 1920 in *Beyond the Pleasure Principle*. Rarely, too, in Freud's popular representations, is his emphasis on the human sexual drive ever given the context of the evolutionary legacy it represented.

But Freud had hoped to establish his work within the parameters of evidence-based science from the beginning. In 1875, as he completed his second year of medicine, he reflected on his yearning for 'a laboratory and free time', and that same year on a summer trip to England it was, as biographer Peter

Gay described it, the 'consistent empiricism' of English scientific books that he admired.[32] He had cut his research teeth on the pure science of marine biology, dissecting eels to test an hypothesis that they were hermaphroditic, unravelling first the nervous systems of fish under the microscope and then the brains of humans.

Fifty-seven years later, having finessed his psychoanalytic theory, he still saw scientific rigour as the benchmark for his research on the human mind: '[psychoanalysis] is a piece of science and can adhere to the scientific world view', he wrote toward the end of his life.[33] In the lead-up to this, he saw himself as being among the positivist scientists, who looked to overthrow the superstitious, mystic, occult traditions of the pre-Enlightenment romantics with mathematics, logic, empirical observation. But it became harder and harder to remain accountable to scientific rigour as he moved away from neurology and toward psychology, which called for giving up the established lingo of neuroanatomy for something entirely unseeable: the part of the mind, Freud believed, responsible for jokes, slips of the tongue, dreams, symptoms and defences – the unconscious.

In 1891, before he had formulated the detail of his hypothesis of the mind, he wrote a seminal paper on aphasia, where a person loses receptive or expressive language, for which he had been studying brain lesions in relation to language apparatus. It was at this point that he came to the conclusion that the study of the psychological, the mind, could not be simply conflated with the physiological, in that it was represented in the brain by dynamic systems: mental function could not be localised.

Facing this conclusion, he abandoned the clinico-anatomical method, which attempted to infer brain function by looking at the way injury to an identifiable part of the brain affected a patient's mind, moving instead to a method that worked on the trained analyst's observations of the patient as a specific individual with subjective experiences. 'Perhaps in the end I may have to learn to content myself with the clinical explanation of the neuroses,' he wrote to his friend Willhelm Fliess.[34]

With that his work moved entirely into the territory we could not see, to put forward hypotheses about this unknown part of our minds. The id was 'a chaos, a cauldron of seething excitement', a soup of primitive and instinctive impulses that sought two goals: sex and aggression, or more broadly life and death (eros and thanatos). This primitive part of our minds, Freud said, which is not accessible to our conscious, wants nothing more than satisfaction of our instinctive impulses: every wishful impulse should be satisfied immediately, regardless of consequence. He said that the conscious part of our minds – the part that experiences the real world, and knows its rules and limitations – feels anxiety when it encounters a situation in which it can't realistically satisfy those impulses. And in a bid to get rid of this unpleasant feeling (for it is always striving for pleasure, according to Freud), it banishes those urges or drives to the unconscious. But! Those driven-away urges remain eternally preserved in our soupy, chaotic cauldron of self, giving off their funk and influence on our conscious behaviours and on our bodies. 'They can only be recognised as belonging to past experience, deprived of their significance, and robbed of their charge of energy, after they have been made conscious by the work of analysis,' Freud said.[35]

His proposed mental machinery existed in an entirely invisible terrain, and the language he used was still situated not far from that of his positivist peers working with the equally invisible matter of neutrons and charges and atoms. Explaining the human tendency to keep their instinctual tensions at an optimal level, he wrote of mental processes as expulsions of energy designed to hold 'constant the mount of excitation' in the 'apparatus'.[36] It extended the idea of the physiologist Ernst Wilhelm von Brücke, who had taught Freud at the University of Vienna, that all natural phenomena are the phenomena of motion. One could easily feel Freud was talking about the mechanics of a centrifuge not the mind of a person.

Even his emphasis on the sexual, the libido, so often used today to frame him as lecherous, had its origins in the pragmatic world of nineteenth-century evolutionary sciences. Though Freud got much wrong in this respect – defending, for example, Lamarckian ideas of specific memories being heritable across generations – his views on the role and development of the sexual drive emerged in the context of serious biological debates of inheritance and natural selection, not from a voyeuristic personal penchant for the lurid, as modern-day caricatures tend to depict.

As a man of science, he was anxious to avoid his work being aligned with the occult. He seemed to worry about being perceived as a charlatan, always pushing against any yearning in himself for the mystical: 'As a young man I felt a strong attraction toward speculation and ruthlessly checked it,' he told his biographer Ernest Jones.[37] When his seminal work *The Interpretation of Dreams* was published in 1899, he pointed out before anyone else could that he was 'against the objections of severe science … [taking] the part of the ancients and of superstition'.[38] And he pushed against any leaning in himself toward philosophy, fearing that reading the great philosophers would lead him to conclusions that would be satisfying but not based on fact. 'I have rejected the study of Nietzsche although – no, because – it was plain that I would find insights in him very similar to psychoanalytic ones.'[39]

Strangely, despite his outward alignment with science, Freud chose as his intellectual confidant the veritable quack Wilhelm Fliess, although the two later became estranged. Fliess was an ear, nose and throat specialist with a penchant for numerology, a belief that humans were governed by biorhythmic cycles of twenty-three and twenty-eight days, and a theory that the nose was the dominating organ of the body. It may be, as Peter Gay has proposed, that from Fliess, Freud could rely on getting sympathy for the criticism he feared receiving from mainstream medicine.[40] He vented to Fliess in 1896, after delivering a lecture on hysteria to the Society for Psychiatry and Neurology, that his colleague

Richard von Krafft-Ebing had said of his hypothesis: 'It sounds like a scientific fairytale.'[41]

And there was something in Freud, too, despite himself, that was lured to the irrational: 'For years he harboured the haunting belief that he was destined to die at the age of 51, and later at 61 or 62 … even the telephone number he was assigned in 1899 – 14362 – became confirmation: he had published *The Interpretation of Dreams* at 43, and the last two digits, he was convinced, were an ominous monition that 62 was indeed to be his life's span,' wrote Gay.[42]

Freud knew that, scientific rationalism aside, he would always be attracted to a kind of mysticism, which he put down to his spiritual Jewish heritage. But he also used his theory of psychoanalysis to uncover meaning behind the displays of superstition he compulsively exhibited: they represented suppressed desires. This was precisely the sort of hypothesis that was impossible to verify.

The writer Janet Malcolm saw in Freud's language a struggle to 'reconcile the unwieldy findings of psychoanalysis with the orderly positivism … in which he had been educated'. In Freud's 1912 paper 'Recommendations to physicians practising psycho-analysis', Malcolm found a distinct inaptness in his analogy of the analyst as a surgeon who must put aside his feelings and work with cold precision, and his description of the state of evenly suspended attention the analyst must achieve: 'the incongruous yoking of the image of the exquisitely relaxed analyst, inclining toward his patient's psyche as a sinuous, long-stemmed plant languorously yields to the law of tropism, with that of the cold, hard surgeon, tensely concentrating his mental forces on the technical job at hand'.[43]

Freud was aware that the nature of his subject, the human mind, posed a threat to his scientific standards, and that the methodical robustness of the evidence he drew on, by nature of the creative language required to express the human story, was weak. He wrote with seeming frustration that his 'case histories read like novellas, and ... lack the serious stamp of scientific method'.[44] He conceived of psychoanalysis as a natural science, in which the mind was no different from any other element of our world that can only be perceived indirectly – a Kantian view that drew on the idea of reality as always being only a representation, never the actual thing. Just as physics or astronomy was based on models of what was observed through measuring devices or telescopes, so was knowing the human mind a matter of observing external perceptions of one's inner state. Freud considered that we have two surfaces with which we perceive the world: the external conscious, which perceives through senses (we see, hear, smell), and the internal, which perceives through feelings (we feel angry, tired, hungry). Both planes of experience, in his view, were part of the physical sciences.

But this reluctance to shape his work on empirical research – objectively observed data gathered through experiments – has been the pyre upon which psychoanalysis has burned. Indeed, philosophers of science have found psychoanalysis to offer the perfect ingredients for modelling how we define pseudo-science – statements or practices that claim to be scientific but are incompatible with the scientific method. Most famously, Karl Popper used psychoanalysis to explain his demarcation theory, which was a way to characterise whether a system of statements can be the concern of empirical science. According to Popper's model, coming up with an hypothesis and proving it was not the key; the system of statements can only belong to empirical science if the statements can be proved wrong, or falsified. Since psychoanalysis offers any number of reasons for a person's emotional make-up, and none can be proved wrong, Popper argued it is a pseudo-science.

For staunch critics that came after Popper, like the Freudian revisionist Frederick Crews, who has written four extensive tomes questioning and then burying entirely the reputation of Freud, there are two pivots upon which Freud's demise turns:

the science, and the man himself. The revisionists paint a picture of a deliberately manipulative fact-fudger with a less-than-clean personal history. There is Frank Sulloway, whose 1979 book *Freud: biologist of the mind* claims that Freud was hardly original in his theory of the unconscious; and worse, that he obscured his influences and the debt he owed to neurobiology, and that his theories drew on already-debunked biological claims. Five years later, philosopher Adolf Grünbaum published *The Foundations of Psychoanalysis*, in which he dissected microscopically Freud's claims of psychoanalysis as a science, declaring it anything but. His formulation was less forgiving than Popper's: it wasn't that Freud had wrongly attempted to make a science out of something that could never be; rather, Freud had assembled bad science. He had made falsifiable predications that had proved false, but had run with them anyway.

Later revisionists Peter Swales and Jeffrey Moussaieff Masson went to forensic lengths to find, in Freud's letters and notes, evidence both of Freud's misrepresentations and his personal dishonesty. Swales put together a case that Freud had been having an affair with his wife's sister, and used this as the basis for a character assassination that worked to cast doubt for many over the substance of any of Freud's writings. Masson's claims ran closer to the bones of psychoanalytic theory itself, hinging on Freud's abandonment of a key hypothesis early in his career. Freud had put forward his 'seduction theory' in the mid-1890s, in which he said that his patients who were suffering hysterical symptoms had brought to him memories that they had repressed of being sexually abused by key male caregivers in their infancy. A few years later, he abandoned this theory, coming to the conclusion that if it ran true then all fathers including his own had been perverse. Instead, he felt it fitted better with what he had proposed about the unconscious mind to say that what his patients had brought him were unconscious struggles they had had as infants, in the form of fantasies (or *phantasies*, as he spelled it, to distinguish it from daydreams), in moving through the various stages of infantile sexuality. Masson, who in the 1980s had access to extensive Freud papers as projects director of the Freud Archives, claimed that Freud changed his theory, eliminating the truth of his patients' actual sexual abuse as children, to serve his own concerns that the abuse stories would be too unpalatable to gain acceptance among his colleagues.

Scientific methodology had mattered to Freud's vision for psychoanalysis, but that may have been his failing. In trying to defend himself against the authority that science represented, he gave himself an impossible task, and by any account he may have been more creative writer than scientist. But in the sphere of the subjective mind, and in a century in which crude lobotomy still seemed a solution to some mental ailments, could science ever have provided a benchmark for Freud's work?

Psychoanalyst Adam Phillips has said: 'I don't think psychoanalysis is a science or should aspire to be one. I don't think it should be a deliberately misleading mystification either, but I don't think these kind of empirical criteria are the only criteria of value. Nobody is going to do empirical research on [the poet] Wallace Stevens.'[45]

Or, as the academic Robert Reynolds put it, to describe the way that psychoanalytic work guesses at a helpful narrative to construct around one's inner life: 'psychoanalysis is the art of speculation'.[46]

How could an act constructed of language ever be held up to science? The German psychotherapist Nini Herman recounted her experience in Jungian, Freudian and Kleinian psychotherapy over almost a quarter of a century, and concluded that: 'The help I sought eventually arrived by the oldest route such salvage operations take: that of one individual's true concern for another in distress.'[47] Her final analyst, in the meaning she made with Herman, broke through to her.

Ψ

Perhaps I too was giving myself an impossible task by looking at my postnatal experience through the lens of Joni's words.

Until I became a mother, I would easily have fitted my analytic experience into 'positive treatment outcome'. Certainly, I had met Freud's markers for fruitful life: *lieben und arbeiten* – love and work. I had arrived at Dr Parkes shortly after my trip to the UK with Gideon, spent in phone boxes calling my family. I had been, after some years on his couch, largely free of anxiety, working productively, living with love. A randomised controlled trial of various versions of me would, I had no doubt, show that the 'me' who ended up with Dr Parkes had the best outcome of all. And yet, things came crashing down.

Had I been indoctrinated into a cult with my reverence for psychoanalytic ideas? I glanced at Noah, who was now engrossed in a segment about an ammonia-free cleaning agent. On the screen, a waxy-skinned man with icy blue eyes demonstrated to a gormless-looking puffy-haired woman how two spritzes of the agent could cut through the thick fat drippings on an iron griddle pan.

Occasionally it appealed to me to reject psychoanalysis as a fiction. For one, it would relieve me of my constant worry about the invisible impact that my postnatal collapse had had on my children. How, if I took psychoanalytic ideas seriously, could it be possible for either child to have made it through their first year of life without some fall-out from my perilous mental state? Would I, despite my efforts to function normally, have communicated to them unconsciously – through the way I held them, the tone of my voice, the look on my face – that I felt I was collapsing? What might it do to a baby to feel that their mother is not on solid ground?

Winnicott said that where the caregiver does not respond adequately or with empathy to the infant's experience of reality, the infant begins to develop an unhealthy false self: 'Other people's expectations can become of overriding importance, overlaying or contradicting the original sense of self, the one connected to the very roots of one's being.'[48] Following Winnicott's theory, a person who develops an unhealthy false self experiences their life with a sense of hollowness, of internal unreality. They develop false relationships, and 'attain a show of being real'.[49] Had I, in the face of my terrible postnatal anxiety, failed to respond to my children with empathy? I was certain I had never neglected them; if anything, I had been overly attentive – perfectionistic about fulfilling their needs. I arranged my day strictly according to when I expected they would want sleep; I breastfed on demand. But was that empathic? If empathy was transplanting oneself under the skin of another's body it seemed now, with distance, that what I had been doing was flailing about in my own body, grabbing onto anything stable in order to escape its crushing need for order, calm, predictability.

I could drive myself mad thinking about the gamma-ray powers of my unconscious intent. Psychoanalytic theory, the idea of us all having desires and motivations that we haven't realised, meant that I might have wounded my children despite myself. What if my postnatal anxiety was all my unrecognised maternal ambivalence bubbling to the surface?

'Mama?' Noah called, his eyes wide, his finger pointing to the TV, to the blackened pan on which a clean silver spot was emerging. 'Dat dirt from children?'

14

'I'm reading about Freud,' I told Aaron.

We were at a reconfigured pottering kiln that was once used to furnace and bake clay dug from eighty metres below ground into ceramics, tiles, chimney pots. It was within walking distance from both his house and Joni's house. The old central kiln, which had been converted into a cafe with gallery, was exhibiting images from biomedical research – complex cell activity intended to be viewed as art. There were startling abstract scenes of fluorescence, synaptic connections shot through with brilliant light. Noah was occupied in the highchair beside me with a croissant that he was transforming into tiny globby balls.

'Ah!' my father replied. 'I read him a long time ago … Dora B, Wolf Man.'

'It's a biography,' I conceded. 'Not the case studies.'

He nodded.

I noticed these days how silver Aaron's hair had gone and it never failed to jar me; the tableau I had of him in my mind's eye was the small black and white passport photo I'd carried around with me since I was seven and we'd moved to Australia without him: masses of dark curly hair, wire-rim aviators. For the year in which he and Paul had remained in South Africa waiting to emigrate I had looked at that photo daily. There had been that brief time after they finally made it to Perth when I'd had him in person, and then Maxine had remarried and she, my stepfather, Joni and I had moved to the other end of Australia, far from Aaron and Paul again. It was only when Reuben was nine months old that Aaron and Paul had moved to be near us. I had missed having my father in physical proximity for twenty-four years. I never said it to him, but there was something reparative for me in the symbolism of the timing; I was nine months when he and my mother had divorced, when I felt he had left me.

'What do you think of Freudian theory?' I asked, jumping straight to it; a croissant would only keep Noah occupied for so long.

I knew Aaron wasn't a Freudian. Hardly anyone was these days. Despite terms like 'Freudian slip' and 'anal' now being in common usage, Freud has fallen distinctly out of favour. Outside of psychoanalytic circles he is often portrayed as either a mad, self-experimenting cocaine user, or a hack, whose claims to the unconscious mind were at best nonsense and at worst dangerous. Within psychoanalytic circles, classic Freudian analysts are rare, if not extinct; the now-mythical thylacine of the profession.

There were two aspects to psychoanalysis – its method and its theory – and each had morphed from its Freudian origins in different ways over the century, with new psychoanalytic subgroups sprouting new languages of reference. There are Jungians, followers of the object-relations analysts like Melanie Klein, and followers of Freud's daughter, Anna Freud, at odds with each other but united in their opposition to followers of John Bowlby. There are the American Ego analysts and the dissident Lacanians. And there are the therapists like Aaron, who have for various reasons not acquired 'analyst' status through the rigorous supervision and five-weekly analysis required to do so, or who eschew strict Freudian method, and are in the branch of therapists known as 'psychodynamic', outside the psychoanalytic circle by technicality. The dolphin of the fish species, if you will. The flow-chart of psychoanalytic factions looks something like a Tokyo subway map, so messy and multiple are its paths.

Freudian or not, all psychoanalysts embrace Freud's radical

concept of our unconscious minds as cauldrons of untapped primitive forces, desires and wishes that bump up against each other, causing us repeated conflicts in our consciously lived lives, and sometimes in our bodies. It was this I was most interested in about Freud's legacy. Is there a part of our brains holding feelings we are not in touch with? Or are we only who we are on the surface, in our conscious thoughts?

'Freud was a genius, but he was *of his time*,' my father answered. 'Nineteenth-century Vienna is a far cry from today.'

Freud's hypotheses about the mind, which changed considerably during the course of his lifetime, can be broadly explained as centring on human sexuality. Our unconscious minds, he said, contain our base sexual desires and instincts, shaping us from infancy. His concept of sexuality was not limited to our genitals, but included all the ways the body could experience pleasure, from the baby's satisfaction at their mother's breast to the satisfaction of a bowel movement.

In infancy, he said, our senses and desires about these bodily experiences, which dominate our existence, are primitive, untethered to social constraints or language. As we move through those stages of psychosexual development he identified that lead to adulthood, these primitive imaginings and feelings are squashed down into our unconscious minds by a mechanism he called 'repression'. With these thoughts and feelings locked away in our unconscious, we can live respectably in society but in the psychic discomfort of unsatisfied wishes, or phantasies, which find symbolic representation in our lived experience, and which we will try as adults to fulfill in ways that confound even ourselves, through our sexual imaginations, our fetishes, our instinctive, inexplicable ways of seeking pleasure and pain, life and death.

But as the writer Janet Malcolm put it, the sexual climate of Freud's time was 'fraught with Ibsenesque gloom and fatalism', with people destined to become either neurotic or hysterical as a result of the abstinence or coitus interruptus necessary to avoid catching gonorrhoea or syphilis.[50] It was worlds apart from our modern era of easily obtained contraception and infinite socially acceptable means to gratify sexual urges, from virtual sex online to legal brothels. This changed context has to be taken into account when considering a Freudian approach to mental suffering.

Freud's views on female sexuality were also gravely limited by nineteenth-century social mores. According to biographer Peter Gay, 'His understanding of women was notoriously inadequate, but he did make great steps beyond what was understood about women when he came on the scene. It was highly unusual in Freud's time even to acknowledge that women had sexual desire.'[51] A significant feminist movement has since developed psychoanalytic theory to encompass and better understand the female experience, including people like Karen Horney, who argued against Freud's idea that female sexuality derives from its lack of maleness, as well as writers and philosophers like Luce Irigaray and Hélène Cixous, who recast mythologies Freud used to describe human development, such as the Oedipus complex, according to the female experience. In feminist psychoanalyst Janet Sayers's rich overview of the key women who have impacted the psychoanalytic movement, *Mothering Psychoanalysis*, she declares: 'Psychoanalysis has been turned upside down. Once patriarchal and phallocentric, it is now almost entirely mother-centred.' By this she is referring to the way that contemporary psychoanalysis is now heavily centred on the maternal–child relationship, through the work of people such as Melanie Klein and Anna Freud.[52]

Aaron continued, now itemising how far we have come in our views of gender and sexuality since nineteenth-century Vienna: 'We've got a biological understanding of gender orientation now that completely debunks Freud's theory of that. And hardly any analysts these days treat their patients with a view of homosexuality as something to be corrected.'

'What?' I interjected. 'He thought homosexuality was correctable?'

'He saw homosexuality as a stage in a person's development. He didn't say that it was a problem to remain in that stage, but he framed it as a stage that in *normal* development a person would move through. It was an arrested development.'

'Wow.' I was a little shocked. 'Didn't this ever make you feel alienated by psychoanalysis?'

Aaron shook his head. 'Homosexuality was not a pathology to Freud. But definitely a lot of the psychoanalytic institutions took his words as though he had said it was. I would have struggled to get my analytic training with the main institutions after I came out.'

I got my phone out and did some googling. The British Psychoanalytic Council had only changed its position on admitting gay and lesbian candidates for training in 2012, I saw. It now states that it 'opposes discrimination on the basis of sexual orientation. It does not accept that a homosexual orientation is evidence of disturbance of the mind or in development.'

'But didn't that upset you, when you read Freud?' While I was waiting for his answer I realised I was sounding like a detective trying to place a suspect at a crime scene, though I wasn't certain what I was hoping to pin on him.

'If I had known I was gay when I first read Freud, I might have felt there was something wrong with me,' he said. 'But by the time I came to terms with my sexuality I had a much better understanding of what he was saying – plus, psychoanalysis has evolved. I must say,' he went on, 'I've never encountered colleagues treating homosexuality as something to be fixed. I never encountered it in my own therapy.'

I was relieved to hear this. The idea of a psychoanalysis that had at its heart the aim of changing a person's sexual orientation was anathema to a process that these days came closest to defining itself as an endeavour to come to terms with reality.

'Freud is dead,' wrote the philosopher and psychoanalyst Jonathan Lear. But, he went on to say, 'it is important not to get stuck on him, like some rigid symptom, either to idolize or to denigrate him. The many attacks on him, even upon psychoanalysis, refuse to recognize that Freud gave birth to a psychoanalytic movement which in myriad ways has moved beyond him.'[53]

Noah was wanting out of the highchair and Aaron was starting to look at his watch. He had walked down to the cafe from his consulting rooms, which were attached to his house. His day ticked over in hour-long increments – the length of a session with a patient plus ten minutes' break, which was the norm for therapists modelling their work on psychoanalytic ideas. Freud had advised 'leasing by the hour' and charging for missed appointments as a way to make the patient motivated to attend.[54] My father, like many contemporary therapists, did not make his patients pay for missed sessions, but he had been influenced by Freud's hour-long model. I had, as long as I could remember, always known that ten minutes to the hour was the time in which my father was likely to answer the phone to me.

'Tell me again about the little girl who wouldn't talk,' I asked Aaron. This was a favourite of mine, a story of a patient he had seen back in Johannesburg in the days when he treated children. The case carried in it for me the magic of the psychoanalytic method, the jolt of a mystery unlocked by a good detective.

'Well, remember, I was working with the theories of the object-relations analysts. They developed a psychoanalytic method that could be used with children. I would observe a child playing, and that's how we would do our work together.'

The analysts Aaron was referring to, like Melanie Klein and Donald Winnicott, had taken Freud's idea of the unconscious in a different direction. The infant's unconscious mind was not busily striving for balance between the life and death drives, in their view, but seeking relationships, and forming unconscious mental representations of themselves in relation to others that would be the blueprints for their interpersonal experiences thereafter.

'I remember. And what happened with the little girl?' I coaxed him on.

'She was about four years old, and what we called a selective mute. She wouldn't talk to her own family. She was a white girl, and it transpired that there were some people she would talk to: anyone with dark skin. She would talk to her nanny, who was Zulu; Xhosa people whom she hardly knew. But never a white person.'

'Not even her own mother or father,' I interjected, knowing the story by heart.

'Yes, that's right. Not even her mother or father. I spent a long time observing her, and listening to her mother talk. And we worked out together, after many months, that the little girl had suffered from a stomach problem as a baby that had caused her chronic pain. She had screamed in agony for much of her first year, and her mother had been so unable to bear the sound that she had given her over, in the heights of her distress and for all her feeds, to the nanny.'

The nanny with dark skin had held her and fed her, and had bore her pain.

'But how did you work that out? Did the mother just say it one day?' I asked.

'No. It was gradual. I had to listen to what the mother wasn't saying too. And I watched the little girl and the ways she organised her play. It was all these little clues, really. It was information from both the little girl's and the mother's unconscious minds, that even they weren't aware of. So then we did a lot of work together to establish the little girl's attachment to her mother, and for the mother to understand her own anxiety.'

'And she began to speak to her parents, the little girl?' I knew the answer but I loved hearing him say it.

'Oh, yes. She did,' he told me.

Before Freud was actually or metaphorically dead, he was working as a neurologist, and his first insight into the idea that a part of our minds unknown to us might be able to affect our conscious selves came about through his mentor, Jean-Martin Charcot, toward the end of the nineteenth century.

While Freud was investigating cerebral paralysis and aphasia in Charcot's department at Paris's Salpêtrière psychiatric hospital, performing microscopic studies of children's brains, Charcot was studying female patients who were experiencing convulsions, trying to distinguish those whose symptoms were to do with brain anatomy and those whose symptoms were psychological or, as it was termed then, hysterical. Psychology was only emerging as a field of science; it had previously been considered part of philosophy. But Charcot was bringing mental states into the field of neuroscience, which had till then only encompassed the organ of the brain in relation to behaviour, and Freud was quickly fascinated by his work.

Observing the women at Salpêtrière, Charcot proposed the idea that hysteria was a genuine mental phenomenon originating in psychic trauma, rather than a performance or exaggeration. He showed how inducing an altered state of mind through hypnosis could reproduce hysteria or remove hysterical symptoms: he could both induce paralysis in someone and cause a person suffering hysterical paralysis to recover. What's more, when the person had recovered, if they were asked to explain their behaviour, they confabulated, or made up an explanation, which indicated they had no conscious awareness of their real motivations.

Also working at Salpêtrière at the time was neurologist Pierre Janet, who was doing a doctoral dissertation in which he outlined a concept of automatism – that a person could undertake an activity without conscious knowledge of their actions because their mind can split into two dissociated consciousnesses. According to Janet, the conscious mind had dissociated from the unconscious mind, which harboured fixed ideas, usually traumatic ones, in relation to the activity. This came close to Freud's later propositions of the unconscious mind, but Janet's more significant influence on Freud was with his theory that people under hypnosis develop, in their altered mind state, a 'magnetic passion' for the hypnotist. When Freud witnessed this same phenomenon taking place in Charcot's hypnosis demonstrations, he gained confidence in his developing idea that strong feeling, in this case between the patient and the hypnotist, could be elicited by parts of the mind one was not aware of. Freud's concept of transference – in which the patient unconsciously projects strong feelings onto the analyst that are a clue to their symptoms – emerged from this idea, and it became a cornerstone of psychoanalytic work: to find out what is going on emotionally between the analyst and the patient that the latter is not consciously aware of.

After Freud's time at Salpêtrière, he heard from his colleague Josef Breuer, who was using hypnosis on a patient named Bertha Pappenheim (known as Anna O in the case studies). Pappenheim experienced strange fits of paralysis, anaesthesia and speech disturbances, sometimes being unable to speak, understand or read her native German. There appeared to be no biological cause for her symptoms. According to Breuer's notes on her treatment she was relieved of the symptoms when, under hypnosis, she articulated certain memories and fantasies. The Anna O case remains controversial as a defining moment in the story of psychoanalysis because it has emerged that she continued to experience her physical symptoms – but it did give her some relief from them. Pappenheim used the term 'the talking cure' for her treatment, and it was she and Breuer in this sense who came upon this way of identifying and treating bodily symptoms that originated in the unconscious mind through talking. It was Freud who, over the coming century, went on to propose the theory and practice of this new field of mind study, departing with Breuer, however, in focusing on infantile sexual conflicts as the source of the unconscious material to be unearthed.

Freud soon gave up hypnosis as a technique, finding that if he simply let the patient say whatever came to mind – free association – they provided useful verbal material quite easily. Nonetheless, hypnosis revealed something hugely significant to his work: it shone a light for him on the psychological laws of mental life. Seeing Charcot demonstrate, through hypnosis, that a range of people – not only women, not only men, and not only those with neurotic or hysterical symptoms – could be instructed to develop a physical ailment, like a paralysis, showed him 'the possibility that there could be powerful mental processes which nevertheless remained hidden from the consciousness of men'.[55] And, what's more, that this state of unconscious enactment was part of the 'familiar phenomena of normal psychological life and of sleep'.[56] Everyone had an unconscious mind.

Aaron had once, reluctantly, hypnotised me. As a teenager, thrilled by the discovery that he had been trained in hypnosis at university, I'd convinced him to try it on me.

I lay, with the reverence of one about to be sacrificed for the higher good, on the bed Aaron and Paul kept pretty for me in my bedroom away from home, the evaporative air-conditioning barely diluting the heat of that Western Australian summer. Aaron held a pencil above me, its tip hovering in the air. I was to look at the dot of its lead point as steadily as I could. He brought it down slowly. I was, he instructed me in a low, even voice, to relax, to keep my eyes on the pencil, let my lids get heavy. Hypnosis relies on the subject's willingness to participate, and my father could not have found himself a more suggestible subject – my arm levitated on his instruction, my fingers numbed when he told them to.

'Do you remember that?' I asked him now.

He laughed. 'You begged me! I can't believe I did it.' He was ashamed of the showman connotations of hypnosis after all these years. *It's not something I do in my work*, he'd said every time I'd nagged him to try it on me. I remembered my arm, inhabited of its own will, and how it had lowered itself back to its position beside me on the bed, and how my father had instructed, in his somnolent bass, that it would begin to go numb, and how it had. When he had approached it with a sewing needle I had not flinched.

'Didn't you stick a pin in my arm?'

He looked surprised. 'Yes, I remember that. The pin thing was to reinforce and confirm the suggestion I had made to you that your arm was numb. Don't forget, the method of hypnosis I was doing is based on an idea of accessing the unconscious mind through suggestion.'

Back in the 1970s, before Aaron moved on to his eventual interest in psychoanalytic therapy, he was completing his master's in psychology, and had been trained in a kind of hypnosis called Ericksonian hypnosis, which uses a technique known as 'paradoxical communication'. Milton Erickson, after whom it was named, was a maverick, prone to adopting rather off-beat strategies in his work with patients to engage what he deemed to be the patient's unconscious mind. He believed that in a deep trance, people have entered a state in which they are responding from a part of their minds they are not aware of – an unconscious part. But his concept of the unconscious was nothing like Freud's hostile construction of self that banished unacceptable thoughts: Erickson said it was a healing force that could effectively produce change if communicated to indirectly or using metaphor, language play and storytelling rather than authoritative command. His prediction was that the person would resist overt direction, but their unconscious mind could be influenced.

'And I think you also told me it wouldn't bleed?' I continued, eager to get to the part that interested me before our time was up.

He looked perplexed. 'Something about it not bleeding rings a bell. But, no, I would have maybe told you it wasn't going to bleed because I wasn't putting it in very deeply; I said it so you wouldn't worry. I wasn't saying the hypnosis would stop it bleeding.'

'Oh,' I said.

Aaron looked at me askance. 'Let's make some time to talk about this. I have to get back to my rooms,' he said, wrestling Noah from the highchair and holding him high, so that Noah let out a joyful squeal.

'[G]reater authorities than I … were in the habit of diagnosing neurasthenia as a brain tumour', Freud once wrote, of the challenges he and his colleagues faced in late-nineteenth-century Vienna in ascertaining whether a patient suffered from a material disease or an emotional disturbance.[57] One thing was certain from the groping in the dark that Freud and his colleagues were doing as they moved between their microscopic brain samples and their quiet rooms of hypnotism and talk: the mind and the body were indivisible.

We grope less in the dark today, armed with the technology to look inside the living brain, but we are hindered by something else: the specialisation of the sciences. Neurology and psychiatry have galvanised into distinct streams of study, and the institutionalisation of each hampers the ways that knowledge passes between the fields – and the interest that specialists take in moving across fields. Nowadays, neurologists stick to diseases of the nervous system, and the 'hysterical' illnesses that fuelled Freud's theory of the mind are considered relics of a bygone era.

According to one group of researchers, those illnesses are as common now as they were in the nineteenth century. 'Conversion' illnesses (as psychiatry now deems them; in neurology they are 'psychosomatic symptoms') remain prevalent. Instead, what has declined is the interest that the medical fraternity and science has taken in these illnesses, as the treatment of the brain and treatment of the mind have moved into disconnected camps, post-Freud: 'The split between neurology and psychiatry, neurological disinterest in hysteria, physician anxiety over misdiagnosis, embarrassment at the excesses of psychological theory and the enthusiasm of patients with conversion symptoms to be told they have a neurological disease are all powerful reasons why hysteria has for so long been resided in a no-man's-land between neurology and psychiatry,' explains a paper by a joint team of clinical neuroscientists and psychiatrists at the University of Edinburgh.[58]

Suzanne O'Sullivan, a neurologist with a keen interest in the mind, confirms this divide in her book *It's All in Your Head: stories from the frontline of psychosomatic illness*, where she reveals the challenges she faced in taking seriously the suffering of patients whose illness had no identifiable biological cause:

> Up to one-third of people seen in an average general neurology clinic have neurological symptoms that cannot be explained and, in those people, an emotional cause is often suspected. It is very difficult for a patient to be given the news that their physical illness may have a psychological cause … And doctors can be reluctant to offer it up, partly for fear of angering their patients but also for fear of what they might have missed. Patients often find themselves trapped in a zone between the worlds of medicine and psychiatry, with neither community taking full responsibility.[59]

It is as though the mind, having invisible borders, cannot stay apace with the body in the great surging forward of medical knowledge.

I phoned Joni from the car on the way home.

'Remember the time Dad hypnotised me? That summer? He made my arm lift and then he stuck a pin into it, and I didn't even feel it?'

My sister laughed. 'I don't think he put the pin in. He just said he was going to put the pin in.'

'But I remember it going in. It was like magic. There was no blood.'

'Magic's right,' she answered. 'There are ways you can do that so that you don't bleed. But it's not the hypnosis; it's a trick.'

'Why would Dad want to trick me?'

Joni hesitated. I could hear the sound of computer keys clacking. 'Here. I've found a clinical trial on the effect of hypnosis on bleeding. It's not very robust' – she gave a sort of chuckle – 'pretty poor, actually … small number of subjects … not much evidence …'

My sister had been there that stifling day, observing the fascinating event. She was seventeen, deeply into Gothicism, clad all in black, with her hair always pulled back severely or let loose wildly around her talcum-white face, headphones in, pounding out some slow dirge or industrial boom or discordant punk. The scene of my hypnotism had suited her macabre interests. Nowadays, her interests were grounded less in cultural movements than in scientific research, and when it came to hypnosis our combined memories of that day amounted to little more than anecdote.

But I wanted proof. I was shaken by the apparent unreliability of my memory, by my wish for the power of my father's actions: that he could affect my body via a part of my mind I did not feel at the helm of. I was the last person to believe in ghosts or spells or magic, so what was this thing I believed in that Joni did not?

15

In Mary Shelley's *Frankenstein*, the young student Victor Frankenstein is determined to apply the natural sciences to the 'deepest mysteries of creation': the capacity to give life to lifeless matter. The tragedy of the monster he ends up giving life to from corpse parts comes about because the monster is not merely animated – given blood that circulates and lungs that breathe – but sentient, conscious, thinking; capable of turning into thought the feeling of the deep rejection of his creator, who ends up abjectly horrified by his own creation. It turns out being alive, in Shelley's vision, comes with having a mind.

But what is it Victor has bestowed on his monster?

'Whence, I often asked myself, did the principle of life proceed?' Victor asks, in the lead-up to his discovery of this force of animation, this *élan vital*, that he uses to bring his tragic monster to life. We, the readers, never find out what this force is. Shelley, cleverly, by feigning a desire to protect us from the fate that befalls Victor, avoids having to come up with an answer for that which, nearly two hundred years later, continues to elude us – the question of what it is that a living, feeling, thinking being is composed of: 'I see by your eagerness, and the wonder and hope which your eyes express, my friend, that you expect to be informed of the secret with which I am acquainted; that cannot be … I will not lead you on, unguarded and ardent as I then was, to your destruction and infallible misery.'[60]

Ψ

Susannah Cahalan was the name of the neurologically ill journalist that I had talked to Joni about; the one whose story had seemed to mirror this philosophical crisis in me about the locus of my postnatal experience. Was it mechanical, organismic, a result of the biochemistry and genes and hormones of my body? Or was it emotional, mental, the result of the part of me that is formed of memories and feelings? Was it my mind or my body first? Both in collusion? There was no test for the origin of suffering. And whether psychoanalysis, the most definitive theory to date of the subjective human mind, and my chosen treatment, had been proven effective according to scientific parameters was not answerable without asking another thing first.

My inquiry boiled down to a far bigger conundrum: What is a mind? What, and where, is this sentient part of our selves that experiences emotion? Where in me lay the *sorrow of fathers leaving* that I had tried to explain to Dr Parkes as the tingling discomfort I felt along my once-broken hand bone?

Cahalan's story bore the complexity of my query: if a woman could exhibit mental symptoms as the result of physical illness, what did this tell us about where, in our selves, our minds or forces of animation lie? Cahalan had called her book, about the month in which she had been so ill, *Brain on Fire*. Though she was nearly institutionalised for her mental symptoms of paranoia, hallucinations and intense mood swings, she was satisfied, by the end of her story, to assign it to the realm of bodily illness: she had a rare disease called anti-NMDA receptor encephalitis: 'there likely was a pathogen of some sort that had invaded my body, a little germ that set everything in motion … maybe it was in something I ate or something that slipped inside me through a tiny wound on my skin …?'[61]

What Victor Frankenstein came up against, in taking modern natural science to the realm of philosophical matters deemed immaterial was what scientists, philosophers, neurologists and psychologists continue to come up against in trying to identify where our very selves lie. The ancient Greeks wrestled with it, Plato and Aristotle, one a philosopher and one a scientist, both speaking of the mind in terms of the soul – an entity separate to the body. In the seventeenth century, philosopher René Descartes' theory of mind–body dualism reigned: the mind and body were distinct, of different matter, the mind outside of regular physics. Descartes failed, though, to explain how the mind, being in this place beyond regular physics, comes to act on the body, though he offered the pineal gland – a part of the brain not bilaterally duplicated, and so in some sense a portal between two realms – as the site where this occurs.

His dualism theory, of humans as imbued with something other than body that he also called 'soul', put a distinction between us and animals, which he believed were more like automata, animated by physical life but void of mental events. After Descartes, philosophers including Spinoza, La Mettrie and Cabanis became famous for their mind-stuff theories, which ran into broader debates over materialism and metaphysics. Spinoza saw the body and mind as two sides of a biological process: 'The object of the idea constituting the human mind is the body,' he wrote. But no one could overcome what Descartes had struggled to explain – the *Cartesian impasse* of how the mind comes to work on the body.

Physiologists and neurologists soon entered the fray and empirical observation began to dominate the scientific method. The story of the mind–body divide moved firmly into an acceptance of the material brain as the organ of the mind, and the focus turned to anatomical investigation. By the eighteenth century, brain studies had moved from the rudimentary (and sometimes socially dangerous: the shape and size of the cranium, according to physiologist Franz Josef Gall, revealed correlating qualities about the cerebrum underneath it, and the mental abilities each possessed) to the highly developed. The nineteenth century saw further development, with, for example, physiologist

Marie-Jean-Pierre Flourens' then groundbreaking surgical lesions of animal brains showing the 'contralateral' nature of brain lobes – that the left hemisphere affects the right side of the body, and vice versa.

Electrical brain stimulation also made an entry around this time with German physiologists Gustav Theodor Fritsch's and Julius Eduard Hitzig's taking to living animals' brains with electrodes and showing in greater detail the way that manipulation of sites on the cortex related to the body's movement. By the turn of the twentieth century, neurology had entered a comparatively nuanced sphere, with clinical observation and autopsy data facilitating more comprehensive theories about the structure of the brain, its interaction with the body and the evolutionary function of this set-up. In France, Paul Pierre Broca identified a language-processing area of the brain after autopsying a man known as 'Tan', who had suffered a brain injury, and who understood language but was only able to say the word 'Tan'. In Germany, Carl Wernicke identified a region of the brain involved in speech comprehension, after seeing the location of lesions on the brain of a man who had been able to speak and hear but unable to understand what was said to him or written words, and, in Austria, Freud's colleague Theodor Meynert put forward an hypothesis of the body as being represented in the cerebral cortex.

It was in the climate of these kinds of discoveries, along with an emerging focus in neuroscience on psychology as a branch of medicine rather than of philosophy, that Freud began to formulate his theory, in which – against the tide of Wernicke and Meynert and Broca and others – he hypothesised that the mind was not located statically in clear regions: it was dynamic, dispersed in the physical, and substantially beyond cognition.

We can watch living brains at work now. Water moving through fibrous tissue will show the connections between areas of the brain as vibrant threads on a diffusion tensor image; oxygen that joins up with glucose to fire our neurons will bruise shadows into the pixels of a functional MRI scan, revealing areas of the brain that are active; radioactive markers expand out into blooms of colour during positron-emission tomography where energy is being burned; and the low-level light waves of near-infrared spectroscopy shone into the brain provide data on its processes. Because these techniques offer such a clear view of deeper parts of the brain and can be used on living humans, the information they provide is vastly superior to autopsy observation or to the relatively crude conclusions drawn from older brain-manipulation techniques that failed to work at a neuronal level (neurons being the working blocks of brain function).

Still, in some ways, as we come closer to knowing we move further from it too. With the expansion of research approaches has come a problem for brain science in the form of a lack of common language. As sociologist Hilary Rose and neuroscientist Steven Rose point out in their wide-ranging book on the claims of the bioscience industry and its promises for a Brave New World, *Genes, Cells and Brains: the Promethean promises of the new biology,* neuroscience does not exist as a single science. It was a term coined in the 1960s to bring together the varied studies of the brain and nervous system: 'Even when ostensibly studying the same subject ... cognitive psychologists, molecular biologists and brain imagers have few points of contact, working with different understandings of the phenomenon they study even when using the same words. Two textbooks on memory, for example, each written by a leading expert in the field, one a molecular biologist, the other a cognitive psychologist, share almost no references in common.'[62]

If you trace the ways scientists and philosophers have approached the notion of an unconscious you see this definitional flux. Western philosophers of the seventeenth century had long-debated theories of the mind that included aspects beyond our awareness. Seventeenth-century philosopher Gottfried Wilhelm Leibniz emphasised the perceptions of which we are not immediately conscious, and the term 'unconscious' was being used already in the first part of the nineteenth century by the German romantic philosophers to denote the concept of 'will'.

In 1911, Swiss neurologist Édouard Claparède demonstrated that we can have thoughts that are beyond our conscious awareness with his pinprick experiment on a woman with Korsakoff's syndrome who was unable to lay down new memories. Each day, he shook the woman's hand in greeting, but one day he hid a pin in his palm and pricked her painfully on greeting. The next day, she refused to shake his hand, although she could not say why.

An idea of a part of our minds working without conscious thought is well embraced in contemporary cognitive neuroscience. The psychologist Karl Lashley noted, in his 1950s work on memory formation, that information-processing happens largely without our awareness, in a non-conscious part of our minds. We only consciously notice the *outcomes* of the work our minds do in our everyday living: the rest stays beyond our awareness. The now-famous case of the patient known as HM – who became amnesic after having his hippocampus removed in the 1950s in a bid to stop his epileptic fits – and the studies that pioneering neuropsychologist Brenda Milner did on him, showed us that we are capable of learning new perceptual and motor skills even when we lack the ability to form new conscious memories. Those perceptual and motor skills are retained beyond our consciousness, in what is now commonly referred to as implicit or procedural memories (our conscious memories for people, objects and places are declarative or explicit memories).

Substantial experimental evidence has shown these different forms of conscious and non-conscious mental knowledges, too; that we can drive from one place to another without any memory of operating the vehicle, or considering directions; and that we can take in stimuli subliminally. If consciousness is a mental state of knowing, you could consider the brains of newborn babies as operating on a non-conscious level: they do not use the area of the brain, the frontal lobes, that is linked to the conscious experience of emotion (this kicks in at around six months). They lack the cognition to consciously know their emotions.

Contemporary experiments on people with brain injuries that have set out to identify the origins of specific bodily functions have shown, too, that one part of the brain is capable of *not knowing* what another part of the brain does know, in fascinating ways. We know, for example, that the brain is composed of two hemispheres, each usually responsible for specific functions, and that the white tissue of the hemispheres, known as the cortex, is joined by a band of fibres called the corpus callosum. The work of neuroscientist Michael Gazzaniga revealed that people who have had their corpus callosum severed through injury or surgery for severe epilepsy (severing it interrupts the spread of seizure activity between the hemispheres) behave as if they have two minds. Because the connections in their neocortex (where language, movement control and conscious thought occur) are severed they may, for example, be unable to identify verbally an object in front of them, but if they feel around in a bag for it they can retrieve it. One part of them knows the object (the part that knows how the object feels and what shape it takes) while another doesn't (the part that puts visual cues to words).

Neuroscientist Antonio Damasio's work has also shown that we store information about our emotional responses implicitly so that it remains in our minds without us consciously knowing it. Only when we become conscious of those emotions, which he sees as part of our internal physiology, do they become what Damasio calls 'feelings'. His well-known study – known as the good guy/bad guy experiment – of a man named David who had suffered brain damage so that he was unable to form memories showed that even without conscious memories we retain emotional experiences. David was given three men to interact with on separate occasions; one who was kind to him, one who was neutral, and one who antagonised him. After some days, he was shown photos of the three men and asked to identify who he would go to for help, and who was his friend. He claimed not to recognise the men or to have seen them before, but in 80 per cent of selections he chose the 'good guy' and never chose the 'bad guy'.

None of these mind models quite align with Freud's division of the psyche to explain the pathological processes of mental life, in which unconscious thought – which has been stripped of its verbal framework, its attachment to language, through the mechanism of self-protective mental work that he called repression – affects our behaviour and conscious psychological state. Freud's most lasting conception of the mind, which changed significantly over the course of his lifetime, encompassed the structures of the id, ego and superego. The id is where his 'unconscious' resided: a part of our minds that is primitive, formed of aggressive and sexual drives, untethered to the rules of language. The ego was the part of our mind in touch with the limitations of reality, and the superego our moral conscience. The three systems of id, ego and superego, he proposed, interact to do the repressing in order to keep us in some sort of equilibrium with our basic strivings toward two opposing things: life and death, pleasure and pain.

The process of talking, free-associating and comprehending the analyst's interpretations, Freud thought, brought language to the primitive drives behind our behaviour and feelings, and in doing so made them conscious, freeing us from their tyrannical effects.

Psychoanalysis has been the most comprehensive intellectual attempt to study the subjective, sentient self – the part of Frankenstein's monster that Victor unwittingly overlooked – and to reframe the concept of the body–mind relationship to give primacy to the effect the mind has on the body, rather than the prevailing nineteenth-century view that mental states were caused by physiology. But without empirical studies, without a concrete physiological discovery of the part of the brain that is the mind, it has never found its place as Freud hoped in the framework of science. Indeed, among scientists it has historically been considered to hover in the no-man's-land of philosophy or, worse, in the trenches of fiction. Still, nothing has ever been as transformative for me as good literature.

Rasputin, the Russian mystic who befriended Tsar Nicholas II at the turn of the twentieth century in St Petersburg, was thought by many then to have used hypnosis to stop the bleeding of the haemophiliac heir Alexis. No one ever saw him hypnotise Alexis, but Rasputin's later interest in the practice, reported by his guards, led many to conclude that this is what he had been doing when he prayed with Alexis during his bleeds, though the first time he allegedly affected Alexis's bleeding came when the little boy was only two and unconscious – hardly an optimal state for being put into a trance.[63] I'd always concluded he must have just had the good fortune of arriving in time for the tsarevitch's bleeding to stop on its own. Luck and illusion.

And yet, something in me very much wanted to believe that my father had been able to do what I was sure Rasputin had faked. It was possible, but nonetheless a repugnant idea to me, that my tight grip on a Freudian theory of the unconscious was necessary for me to maintain a belief in Aaron's good intentions. A defence, as Freud would say, if I were to believe him.

There was one group of researchers focusing on Freud's construction of the mind: they called themselves *neuropsychoanalysts.* When I heard this name I could only imagine a kind of interspecies professional: bearded men in white coats operating microscopes awkwardly from a prone position on plaid chaise longues; frizzy-haired women with interesting brooches marking rat behaviour on charts.

The founder of the neuropsychoanalysts was from my birthplace, South Africa. His name was Mark Solms. Google revealed a man always behind a lectern or holding a model of a brain, but bearing other signifiers that betrayed those symbols of stagnant academia: rolled-up shirtsleeves, wild hair, a glass of wine in his hand. He had a vast body of published articles to his name, on topics ranging from the brain mechanisms of dreaming to the application of psychoanalytic methods to understanding complex neuropsychiatric phenomena, such as anosognosia, where a person does not seem aware of their own brain damage. In one article, written for the British Psychological Society, Solms explained the aim of neuropsychoanalysis as being 'to introduce the psyche into neuropsychology – to demonstrate that the brain cannot possibly be understood if the subjective aspect of its nature is neglected or even ignored'.[64]

To understand the origins of neuropsychoanalysis, according to Solms in his book *The Feeling Brain*, you have to revisit Freud and those matters that vexed the long trail of mind–body theorists over time.[65] Freud was a monist – he considered that the mind and the brain were of the same material. Though he began his investigations of the mind using the only method possible at the time, the clinico-anatomical approach (observing how a person's mind changed after brain damage to a specific site), he soon felt its limitations. The dynamic mind that he had begun to conceive of, complex in its connectivity and dispersed through various substrates of the brain, was, drawing on the work of the philosopher Immanuel Kant, not *in itself* something a person could perceive directly but, rather, it made itself consciously known through the act of feeling. Feelings, then, were what needed to be studied to know the mind, in the way that any other component of nature should be studied to reveal its workings.

The way forward was to develop a method of studying feelings through clinical work with patients, and then to draw from that work a comprehensive theory: his psychoanalysis.

Neuropsychoanalysis, which is a term coined by Solms, defines a number of threads of inquiry and research that straddle both the neuroscientific and the psychoanalytic shores. Just one of the threads, if you follow it back, is the one that Freud let go of when he abandoned the clinico-anatomical method: the study of brain-injured patients and their minds in order to come to a comprehensive map of human mental apparatus. As Solms explains in *The Feeling Brain*, he and his colleagues believe technological and methodological advancements in neuroscience, developments in affective neuroscience (the study of the neural mechanisms of emotion) and in the study of animal behaviour in the areas of attachment, separation and loss, now compel science to take Freud's work further than it was able to go during his time.

All the threads of neuropsychoanalytic study take as their central research motivation what had been at the heart of Freud's thinking: that the mind is a material part of nature able to be studied scientifically, with only one important quality that causes it to be different from any other part of nature: it is an object and it is also a subject. It can not only be perceived as a thing contained in the material of the brain; it, itself, feels, and those feelings are viable material for study.[66] Neuroscience has studied it as an object, and psychoanalysis has studied it as a subject, and neuropsychoanalysis seeks to make links between those two aspects of it, declaring that it is not one or the other: it is *both*.

There is relief to be found in locating illness in the corporeal. In recent years the concerted push from mental health advocates to treat mental illness as you would bodily illness has had a necessary effect on reducing stigma: we don't blame people for physical illness, so why blame them for mental illness? This is inarguably true; neither should accrue blame. And nor should the mind be blamed for the physical – *You can beat your cancer if you think good thoughts*; *You should see a psychologist for your endometriosis*, et cetera. Psychoanalysis has, at its darkest moments, caused untold suffering to people with treatable physical diseases who were told it was all in their minds. A Freudian influence on American medical sciences in the 1930s, for example, saw ulcerative colitis treated as a psychosomatic illness, after a Columbia University medical student published an article in the *American Journal of Medical Sciences* in which he claimed to have found common psychological traits among twelve ulcerative colitis patients. The resulting experimental treatments included psychotherapy and horrific physical interventions like lobotomies.[67]

But if we consider the mental as also bodily does that mean it is best treated medically? What if we start to understand that words, talking, relating, thought, come from the biological too? What is immaterial arises from the material. Our bodies are affected at a basic cellular level by both chemical intervention and by living and speaking and understanding. Unless you are a pure dualist, unless you think that our selves exist on a supernatural plane like spirits or ghosts, what else can thought be but a product of our neurons, or some other physical matter perhaps of such a quantum scale that we are yet to know it?

Neuropsychoanalysis seemed to be taking this biological approach to mind as its central project. The organisation had an annual congress, and the next one was in Holland. I checked the dates. It was the week before Gideon was due to go to England for work. He had been trying to convince me to make it a family trip. It seemed fated.

I phoned Aaron.

'How would you like to go with me to a conference in Holland in two months?'

16

In Dr Parkes's consulting rooms all my questions of biology and evidence and brain science returned to their academic pedestals. Twice a week, I lay on his couch and recounted my dreams, said whatever, cried. Twice a week I was silent, said nothing at all. Outside those doors life was a freefall of growth – one white molar pushing up through pink gum, size 1 clothes bagged and packed away, no more swaddling, cot lowered, safety locks back on cupboard doors, a shoe grown too small. Inside, there is no way to describe what went on.

I dreamed over and over again of a city in Europe that I had been to and wanted to visit again, that was near-magical in its exotic delights: it was filled with hanging lanterns, a warm yellow light, the smell of baking bread, the smoke of cooking. It was Granada, where I had been as a young adult on my year-long backpacking trip, and Berlin, which I had only read about. It was the upcoming time in Holland. It was Paris, again, but this time with pleasure.

What was it I gained in that room? What was it in there and with Dr Parkes that could lift me from feeling there was nothing to salvage in myself, that I would always be trying to go overseas as I had as a teenager, never able to leave home? If the European city I dreamed of was the life I wished to live, autonomous, creative, resilient, adult, it beckoned closer every time I returned to Dr Parkes.

'You're benefiting from a good therapeutic alliance,' Joni told me. The concept of therapeutic alliance refers to the quality of the relationship between the therapist and patient, the strength of their collaboration, and the way their goals line up for outcomes. Studies have shown that the weight of these factors determines how successful therapy will be, regardless of the method or mode of therapy itself. In Joni's version of things, any progress I was making with Dr Parkes was because we both wanted the same thing: for me to feel better, or to know what made me feel bad. The validity of Freud's model of the mind was irrelevant.

Was she right? Would I have made exactly the same progress, fallen into exactly the same panic, understood myself any more or less if I had gone twice a week to see a cognitive behavioural therapist, who would have given me exercises to change my unhealthy conscious thoughts, or to a counsellor, who would have offered me concrete, real-life advice about how to manage my problems? Maybe I would have made the same progress visiting the psychiatrist once in a while to report back on my feelings and tweak my medication.

Joni had in recent years undergone cognitive behavioural therapy (CBT), which had amounted to a veritable familial rebellion at the time. Aaron and I had shaken our heads gravely at each other at any furtive opportunity during family gatherings when Joni had mentioned how it was going. When she had undertaken a kind of exposure treatment for her fear of flying that involved learning about the workings of aeroplanes and then sitting in one and then taking a flight, we'd had sceptical phone conversations about it.

'It'll be a short-term fix. The fear of flying represents something else, I've got no doubt,' my father said.

'It'll transmute. She'll get scared of heights,' I'd proposed.

It was relatively easy to assess whether a course of CBT helped with a specific concern, like being able to get onto an aeroplane without having a panic attack, but when it came to psychoanalysis, a long-term, deeply interpersonal treatment that might not necessarily have a clear symptom to address, it was trickier.

Psychoanalysis, both as a theory of the structure of the mind and as a form of treatment, is constantly evolving. At a micro level, the evolution is cultural and contextual; for example, in recognising how outdated Freud's views on women were, working as he was in pre-emancipated old world Europe. The majority of analysts nowadays also work more loosely with his frameworks of human dynamics and the ways he thought we move through psychosexual development. The Oedipus complex, for example – in which he proposed that the male child harbours unconsciously a wish to kill their father in order to take up the position of the primary love of their mothers, and that they must resolve this wish by coming to accept the bounds of reality and eventually by identifying with their father – might be, for the contemporary analyst, an appreciation that at some point in an infant's life they must face the challenge of negotiating a third person's presence in the dyad between them and their primary carer, and find a way to accept the disappointment and envy they feel about this.

On a more macro level, as a whole field, psychoanalysis tends to have moved away from focusing on the Freudian notion of drives and toward the work of later object-relations theorists. They still draw broadly on Freud's work in taking as their central tenet the idea of a dynamic unconscious mind that battles its own conflicts beyond conscious awareness, but the conflicts are rooted less in Freud's biologically influenced sexual and aggressive drives than in the internalised patterns of a person's early care and relations with their early caregivers.

As an example, the contemporary psychoanalyst Neville Symington (making reference to the language of founding object-relations analyst Melanie Klein) explained the analytic experience in this way:

> the patient transfers on to the analyst responsibility for emotional development in a failed area. One aspect of this process is that the patient needs to transfer on to the analyst his or her bad inner objects; the other aspect is that the patient requires an emotional capacity in the analyst in the particular area where there has been developmental failure. It is for this reason that the transference is the central locus of cure. It is also the instrument through which the analyst arrives at an understanding of his patient, which is what essentially differentiates psychoanalysis from counselling or other therapies.[68]

You can see in this description how Freud's legacy lingers in one sense (the notion of transference and the notion of an inner life needing decoding), but in another is replaced by the language of object relations.

Analytic patients rarely know outright the therapeutic framework their analyst is using. 'We all read Freud,' Aaron had told me when I'd asked him if he drew on Freudian theory in his work. 'And we read Jung, Klein. For me, it's Bion. You go with what makes sense to you.' At the time, hearing him list off some of the many analytic greats to choose from, I had imagined Joni's ire: *Should a person have to become familiar with all the various theoretical approaches to choose the best kind for themselves? That's what evidence-based science is about: eliminating what doesn't work.*

I hadn't needed Joni's voice in my head saying these things. I had shouted them myself at Dr Parkes frequently. 'I don't even know what theory you are applying to me! Is that Kleinian? I have no idea of the basis of our work together!' I had, as was my pattern, found Dr Parkes through my father's recommendation, and had been in such crisis at the time I began our work together that I had never thought to ask what sort of psychoanalyst he considered himself to be or, for that matter, whether psychoanalysts worked with one kind of theory or many. From time to time I'd had those bursts of rage toward him in which I demanded to know which school of analysis he was drawing on, and he had called my attention to my need to view him as the bearer of some kind of authority. Later, I came to understand that contemporary analysts don't necessarily work with only one theoretical framework in mind. And sometimes they adjust their theoretical framework to attend to the specific needs of the person in front of them. 'I am working with you, and the question of your theoretical framework. What theory do you live by?' he said to me one day. 'That seems to me more relevant than what mine is. But if you want to know what we are doing here, we are trying to understand your problem, and I am doing that by looking both at what you say and what you don't say.'

This reminded me of what the psychoanalyst Adam Phillips said:

> [You're trying to] discover what the patient's cure would be … what would it be to live better as themselves … and there's a conversation and/or an argument, and an ongoing exchange about that … I'm interested in the person's unconscious repertoire of risks, and the reasons for the risks not taken. You're trying to work out what's stopping you enjoying each other's company … that doesn't mean pleasing each other but feeling the company is worth having, and so all the ways one is warding off exchange – those are worth knowing about.[69]

I suspected Dr Parkes had in mind Bion, who railed against such searches for single truths, and for whom pure self-expression was 'to prevent someone who *knows* from filling the empty space'.[70] A few months before his death, Bion had made a recording in which he said: 'I am always hearing – as I always have done – that I am a Kleinian, that I am crazy; or that I am not a Kleinian, or not a psychoanalyst. Is it possible to be interested in that sort of dispute? I find it very difficult to see how this could possibly be relevant against the background of the struggle of the human being to emerge from barbarism and a purely animal existence, to something one could call a civilised society.'[71]

The writer Janet Malcolm identified the variety of theory in the field, and the patient's inherent ignorance of their analyst's theoretical position, as a problem for psychoanalysis:

> Whether an analyst views a patient's immutable silence, for example, as a 'regressive defense' against castration anxiety or sees it as a reenactment of infant trauma will make an enormous difference to the patient ... a great many versions of the truth, couched in great varieties of language and emotional gesture, are being offered in today's analytic consultation rooms to patients who have little inkling of the implications (for themselves) of where their analyst stands on issues of which they have never heard.[72]

The further I got into our work together the more I felt that what we were doing was beyond the bounds of one particular theory. That it didn't matter if Dr Parkes was working in the language of Freud or Klein, or Bion. The effect was, as humanistic psychologist Carl Rogers described, in the experience of sifting through one's unconscious world in the setting of an authentic relationship: 'I launch myself into the relationship having a hypothesis, or a faith, that my liking, my confidence, and my understanding of the other person's inner world, will lead to a significant process of becoming. I enter the relationship not as a scientist, not as a physician who can accurately diagnose and cure, but as a person, entering into a personal relationship.'[73]

Symington makes a compelling case in his book *A Healing Conversation* for analysts to attend to the psychic pain of the individual by considering not the restricted models of 'the official psychoanalytic "textbooks"' but rather the 'features of human life that are at once private and personal and also interpersonal and inherent in all cultures and historical periods'. A patient might be better transformed when the analyst speaks words that 'fit with the emotional behaviour', and those might be words, according to Symington, drawn from literature – from *Middlemarch*, is his example: that 'it drives someone mad if she is not able to love' – rather than from a Freudian textbook.[74]

There were, of course, features that made what I did with Dr Parkes psychoanalysis and not something else; not friendship. First, there was our focus on my feelings *about and toward him* over and above any other material I brought to him. What Freud called the transference: the way I projected my unconscious inner experience onto my relationship with him. It was in those feelings – in the way, he had noted, that I resisted getting wildly angry with him, in the way I felt sure if he did not come to the door within a minute of my bell-ring that he had died, in the way I became despondent and anxious when he went away for a holiday – that I had come to know and recognise how difficult I found separation.

Tied in with this was, more broadly, our attendance to my inner world, or the unconscious material I communicated: my fleeting thoughts, dreams, the way my body felt and expressed itself. The focus always remained on these communications. If, for example, I brought a memory to him about being mistreated by a teacher, he would not begin to advise me about responding to bad-tempered teachers; rather, he might note something about my voice, or my way of holding my body, or my choice of words that might link up to what he knew about me and the ways I repeatedly experienced my relationships, and that would shed light on what this difficult-teacher memory might mean for me.

Some understandings between us I only worked out after the fact. For example, that we were working toward agency over myself, and to uncovering how I defended myself against pain; that it was unhelpful to this task to have him provide bandaids to my needs. That he would not prescribe me medication or hug me. One day I arrived and as I lay down on the couch I said:

'I have the worst headache. I've had one constantly for days. I don't know why.'

'Oh dear,' he responded, quickly moving on to say, 'I am afraid I need to change next week's time.'

We negotiated a new time, and then he moved back to address what I had said as I arrived, offering interpretations on the idea of a recurrent headache. It was often this kind of discussion, in which he drew together what could seem to be disparate things I had said, in which I became quite resistant to the process. 'I have had headaches because I have been working solidly at my computer for a week and my neck is stiff,' I told him with aggravation.

'Then why did you start the session saying that you don't know why you have had constant headaches?'

I cracked my knuckles. 'I was just saying what one says when one wants sympathy.'

'I am not here to give you sympathy,' he answered. 'I am here to help you understand.'

I was silent for a while, processing his train of thought. There had been so many times I had wanted him to hug me, give me a tissue, tuck me under the blanket that sat at the end of the couch.

Then I remembered what he had said when I had told him of my headache. 'But you did give me sympathy! You said *Oh dear.*'

'Did I? Well, I do apologise for that,' he answered, without an ounce of humour.

And there were particular parameters around our work together that gave it a safe shape, that made it somewhere in which I would come to feel I could bring anything I needed to of myself. These were best known in the field as 'containment'. In Freud's work, containment came in the way the analyst's interpretations of the patient's strong transference feelings allowed them to be brought to consciousness through words, and not acted out. His work with a patient called Dora is often considered an example of his failure to do this – Dora's transference toward Freud was so powerfully negative (a re-enactment of the bad feelings she had toward her own father) that in the end she quit analysis.

Bion explained containment as a feature of the analyst's way of relating to the patient that holds the patient's anxieties, much as the mother takes in and holds her baby's anxieties. In Elyn Saks's memoir *The Centre Cannot Hold*, Saks, who had been given a diagnosis of schizophrenia, describes how she felt her analyst provided a space where she could break down into a psychotic state safely:

> For two straight years, I did my work, met my obligations, made it through the day as best I could, and then fled to Mrs Jones, where I promptly took the chains off my heart and fell apart … Mrs Jones had been the glue that held me together … She had been the tether that held me to the outside world, the repository for my darkest thoughts, the person who tolerated all the bad and evil that lay within me, and never judged … knowing I would see Mrs Jones each day helped me contain my psychotic thoughts when I was with other people.[75]

Containment with Dr Parkes also came about in the boundaries we had agreed upon for the work we did together. Freud had set out many of the elements of the psychoanalytic setting that provided these boundaries, and many were commonsense ways of bringing about consistency for the patient, but they had another important function for psychoanalytic work: since my feelings toward him, or the transference, were a primary source of insight into our work together, the regularity and consistency of the frame of our work together was essential. My appointment times were fixed (altering them could be negotiated once in a while for emergencies but it was expected that they would remain on the set time and day, even public holidays); the location did not change; the length of our time together did not change. This gave us important ground rules against which we could both measure our expectations, and with which Dr Parkes could come to understand my reactions better. If, for example, I could not expect to attend my appointment at a specific time each week, and instead we scheduled it in as each week approached wherever it fit in for us both, it would deny us the opportunity to understand my response – say, of disappointment or anger – if Dr Parkes changed our set appointment time one week.

Often I grew frustrated with Dr Parkes for what I called 'putting a psychoanalytic paradigm' on my inner world. Why did he sound like a Freudian textbook, coaxing me to make associations where I felt I had nothing to say?

'Sometimes a cigar is just a cigar,' I yelled at him one day, an apocryphal phrase always attributed to Freud himself.

I had put up great resistance throughout my analysis to the notion that my own central drives came down to eros and thanatos: sex and death (or aggression, as thanatos was often taken to mean). Mostly, even though I understood psychoanalytic terminology more than the average person, my resistance took the form of a fairly stubborn literalness. 'What do you think the snake in that dream represents?' he asked me one day, after I told him of a terrifying python dream.

'I am not going to say penis. I refuse to say penis. You want me to say penis!' I exclaimed.

'I don't want you to say anything,' he responded evenly.

The idea of those drives being at the centre of my self seemed so far removed from my life. *Where in my day of kindergarten drop-offs and cooking and working and wiping noses do I have a window for thoughts of penises?* I would wonder angrily to myself.

And even though I was willingly in a kind of therapy that asked me to pay attention to what I was not feeling consciously, I often refused to accept any feeling in myself unless it was screaming its intent quite obviously.

But my literalness was my very resistance. Eros was not as concrete as penises. It was life. It was hunger and sensuality and love; it was the touch of Noah or Reuben as much as the touch of Gideon. Thanatos was not literally a wish to die. It was all the ways I sought to destroy or to hinder my own growth. It was the ways my anxiety inhibited my living the fully creative and generative life I felt I wished for consciously. Anxiety stopped me feeling hunger; it numbed my sexuality; it gave me writer's block. It stopped me existing as a grown-up woman in the world. In symbolic terms, it stopped me leaving my mother's bed.

'In psycho-analysis there has existed from the very first an inseparable bond between cure and research. Knowledge brought therapeutic success. It was impossible to treat a patient without learning something new; it was impossible to gain fresh insight without perceiving its beneficent results,' wrote Freud in 1926.[76]

This bond was what became known as Freud's *junktim theory*: that there was a unique tie between research and patient outcome in psychoanalysis, so that the process would reveal the theory of how it worked. Only the therapist themselves, based on their unique knowledge of the patient in the psychoanalytic setting, can assess the quality of the experience. Which is, of course, eminently unsatisfactory to empirical scientists.

Nowadays, while clinical work is still considered an essential tool for teaching and grasping psychoanalytic theory, there has been a push from within toward adding a strong core of evidence-based knowledge to the field.

There has also been a push to bring together in one place, for medical practitioners and the public, the evidence of whether psychodynamic therapy works, full stop, for which there is certainly no dearth of research papers. Since as far back as 1917, there have been studies verifying its success, but they have varied so extensively in their parameters, criteria and standards that they have cumulatively failed to stand as useful evidence. They have also, true to the nature of the field's notoriously multiple branches of theory, struggled to offer a unified evidence base across factions.

Previous literature reviews have attempted to bring together this evidence, such as Jonathan Shedler's 2010 paper, in which his analysis of the research led him to conclude that psychodynamic therapy has an equal positive impact on patients as other therapies, such as cognitive behavioural therapy, and that it imparts long-term improvements that continue after treatment.[77] Another paper, from 2014, put out by the Psychotherapy and Counselling Federation of Australia called 'The effectiveness of psychoanalysis and psychoanalytic psychotherapy', conducted a literature review of recent international and Australian research and concluded that: 'Evidence is building … that short- and long-term psychoanalytic/psychodynamic psychotherapies are effective for treating a broad range of mental health conditions. Tentative support is also available for psychoanalysis as effective in the treatment of these conditions.'

Part of the problem with banding together evidence for whether psychodynamic modes of therapy work lies in the notion of what makes a *good outcome* in the first place. Will it always feel good to know the truth? Will it always feel good to come to terms with reality? Adam Phillips puts it this way: 'I'm not interested in outcomes. The point about analysis is it's an anti-commodity. It guarantees nothing … It has to be taken on as a risk … It may make your life worse or better, but it may make your life better by being worse … as in, you might suffer more but feel realer.'[78]

In 1999, the International Psychoanalytic Association's first *Open Door Review* was published, bringing together empirical psychoanalytic treatment research to form a central source of information and a comprehensive evidence base for whether psychodynamic therapy works, defining 'outcome' as *the changes that came about in the patient* and 'process' as *the mechanisms that produced those changes.*

In 2015 it entered its third edition, a 411-page document bursting with studies, discussions and position statements. What is clear from the 2015 *Review* is that psychoanalysis is embracing the variety within its own theories, treatments, bodies of knowledge and research, as well as the irresolvable tension of its place in relation to science:

> In today's knowledge-societies – in which scientific experts compete at all levels for authenticity and credibility … it has to assert itself as a specific, irreplaceable, effective and productive clinical method of treatment and a theory of mind and culture. Through its specific research method, the developing of unique and effective forms of short-term and long-term treatments, by interesting and innovative explanations for the complex phenomenon of individuals and groups as well as of society, psychoanalysis may even increase its public attractiveness as a 'specific science of the unconscious'.

The *Open Door Review* is the most comprehensive attempt to date to draw all the various studies together. In his foreword to the *Review*, Peter Fonagy, outgoing chair of the research committee behind the publication, writes that psychoanalysis now exists in a radically different world in which major advances have taken place in biology and psychology – in the sciences of mental health and in the development of relatively effective approaches to mental disorders that used to only be treated psychoanalytically. At the same time, within the psychoanalytic field, he says, there are ominous signs of stagnancy: 'We are no longer accumulating knowledge – but rather … we are all developing the discipline in our own individual directions.'[79] Fonagy believes there is a 'fragmentation and confusing absence of shared assumptions' among psychoanalysts that is splintering the field to its own detriment. No longer is there enough unity among the various factions to give psychoanalysis the institutional coherence needed to move forward as a field.

And, no, Fonagy does not consider psychoanalysis, as it stands, to be a science: 'It simply does not meet any of the major canons for such activity ... the question is more usefully framed in terms of our vision for psychoanalysis. Should we aim to modify it so it might be more acceptable to the community of scholars who call themselves scientists? Or should we be content to continue to occupy a middle ground between art and science, that we currently inhabit?'

His answer: it might be helpful to the field to adopt an 'attitude or culture which characterises science'. One of the ways this might be done, he suggests, in light of the hurdles of empirically validating psychoanalytic theory (*How can researchers possibly limit the variables that come about in an interaction that involves the private, the complex, the abstract?* he asks) is to bring together evidence from psychoanalytic clinical work with evidence from multiple other data sources: 'experimental, behavioural, epidemiological, biological, etc'.

Specifically, Fonagy says, biological psychiatry must come into the psychoanalytic understanding of the mind, which, in the end, 'reflects functions of the brain'. Fonagy's research interests reflect this approach. In 2009, with collaborators Montague and Strathearn, he identified potential neural actions that point to patterns of parental attachment being transmitted transgenerationally.[80] A biological account of the mind invariably comes down to genes, he says, which are modified by social, environmental and behavioural factors: 'The outstanding two-fold question is how biological processes modulate mental events and how biological structure is modulated by social factors. It is in answering the second of these questions that a scientific psychoanalysis has a clear role to play.'[81]

In saying this, he draws on the compelling case put forward by neuroscientist Eric Kandel in 1999 in the *American Journal of Psychiatry* for psychoanalysis to link up with biology.[82] To leave it in the field of hermeneutics, where it is studied only in words, text, communications, according to Kandel, hinders it 'from continuing to grow intellectually'.

But the tension between the criteria and aims of the hard sciences and those of psychoanalysis endures. Many within the field – most vocally, a group of French analysts, frequently represented by Roger Perron – believe the demands of empirical science ('observability of the phenomena on the part of experienced observers, use of quantification procedures, repeatability of observations, possibility of predicting the occurrence of specific events, falsifiability, use of a non-ambiguous terminology') stand fundamentally in contrast to the aims of psychoanalysis.[83]

In 2006, Perron entered into a published debate in the *International Journal of Psychoanalysis* with another psychoanalyst, Otto Kernberg, about the nature of research in the field.[84] Kernberg believed the field had a 'social responsibility to reassure the public regarding the effectiveness of analytic work ... without [which] we run the risk of being discarded by the mental health delivery systems'. Accomplishing this would involve, he said, linking up with neurobiology, the humanities and social sciences.

But for Perron, psychoanalysis fails at its own task if it tries to apply a unified model to the individual, or curtails the spontaneous expression of the unconscious material that will arise and provide the material for their therapy, which objective scientific models threaten to do.

Mark Solms, it turned out, was the new chair of the research committee behind the *Open Door Review*. The neuropsychoanalysts were definitely moving in on of all this. Holland beckoned to me with answers.

17

'Your grandmother Fay had severe postnatal depression,' my mother told me. We were in my car, on our way to collect Reuben from kindergarten, Noah in the back.

Maxine, too, had moved to Melbourne a few months earlier, and was now living a short walk from us. We could never stay too far from each other. Aaron and Paul and Maxine, Joni and her husband, and me and Gideon and Reuben and Noah now met every Friday night for a traditional yet atheist Shabbat dinner, usually Malaysian takeout eaten by the flickering light of the Sabbath candles. I marvelled often that we had ended up so firmly in each other's lives, so accessible, and at the ways we fitted together as a family: Maxine laughing with Aaron at something that was in the news the day before; Paul, who wasn't in fact Jewish, arriving most Friday nights with the challah bread for the table.

I had not heard this story from Maxine before. My mother delights in remembering her family narrative, even its scandals and shames. She has a gift for raising banal anecdotes and minor infractions to the heights of comic drama, and sensory detail is never spared: aunts who had ankles like thick wurst, distant cousins with fairytale beauty and no morals. But her wit, I knew, belied family truths that were often so painful, so dark, that only humour could tether them to spoken word.

My mother was the youngest, born two-and-a-half years after her sister Lorrie. 'After Lorrie was born,' she told me now, 'Fay became very depressed and was terrified that she would harm her. She might have had postnatal psychosis. She went to see a therapist and went onto medication then.'

Though Maxine was the youngest, Fay had always burdened her with knowledge beyond her years. When Maxine was only three, Fay told her of the feelings she'd had after Lorrie was born. She told my mother this again many times.

'What do you mean she told you this?' I asked. I spoke softly, in case Noah heard us, always worried about the effect my words might have on my children. Some fossilised, pre-verbal knowledge of the damage done by my grandmother's words was lodged inside me.

'She told me lots of things she shouldn't have. She told me she nearly died during my birth. She'd lift up her top to show me the scar that ran down her stomach, like Lady Macbeth's blood stains,' my mother said. While she said this she was lifting her own top, giving herself a dose of insulin, pinching an inch of fat on her abdomen to inject into. It made me nervous when she did this in the car. When I was a child she would inject in her thigh; always a plum bruise fading to yellow there.

Maxine had told me that, after Fay's postnatal experience with Lorrie, Fay had not wanted to have another child, but that Fay's husband, my grandfather Harvey, had. Fay was haunted by grief at what she interpreted as her profound rejection of Lorrie, and she came to believe that she had damaged her irreparably. She became hyper-vigilant about Lorrie, always worried she would hurt herself, likely projecting her own fear of injuring her firstborn.

And then, finally pregnant with my mother, Fay had become terrified she herself would die in childbirth. She was diagnosed with placenta praevia at seven months, and her panic about dying intensified. Eventually, she saw a surgeon who convinced her he would safely deliver her baby by caesarean.

'So did she? Nearly die, I mean?' I asked Maxine.

'No. I was born and we were both fine. But I grew up from a very young age aware that she had not wanted me. She never considered breastfeeding me. She gave me over to hired nurses. When I was three months old, she and Harvey went away on holiday without me.'

It was hard to imagine my grandmother like this. She had, in my memory, been offbeat, wickedly funny, fiercely intelligent. She had been a classic beauty in her youth – a ballet teacher with an hourglass figure, dark hair, a sensuous gap in her teeth. She had abhorred the ravages of ageing. I once got into the lift with her and an elderly man at the old-age home where she ended up in her seventies, and she yelled to me: 'Tell the *meshuganeh* [a Yiddish term meaning *crazy person*] to press three.' Until we had left for Australia, I had been close to her. She was a sort of irreverent co-conspirator in my childhood landscape. She chain-smoked, offered us cigarettes, to our horror. She paid us by the cent to pull out her grey hairs, and cackled wildly at anything mildly amusing that we did. And she was loving – adoring, even – of my sister and me. But the mother I was hearing about feared the depths of her own distress, was painfully involved with her own paranoias, which she failed to keep from her children.

'Was she psychologically insightful?' I asked Maxine.

'She was very concerned to understand herself, to understand why she had felt as she had after Lorrie. She was never given sound information to help her understand that the experience wasn't unique to her. That so many women who experience severe postpartum depression, or psychosis, fear harming their baby. She wasn't offered time at a mother–baby facility, which is so important for a mother to attach to their baby as they emerge from the illness.'

'So what kind of help did she get?' I asked.

'Well, she was full of strange contradictions. She was terrified of doctors but she was happy to be medicated. She was highly intelligent and well-read, but had all sorts of strange medical misbeliefs. After she had me she went to see a psychiatrist – Dr Horwitz, his name was. The best psychiatrist in Johannesburg.

He was a psychoanalyst, actually. She saw him for years, and would come home from her sessions in a rage. It was a horrible time. He put her on Valium and Ativan, and she took them all – more than she should have – and spent the rest of her life on a cocktail of medication.'

Maxine had told me before that she had felt her sister Lorrie had occupied her parents' minds more than she had. That they were always worried about Lorrie, attending to her, while Maxine was assumed to be able to cope without attention, to be capable beyond her years.

'Actually,' she told me now, 'Granny Fay told me that I had been born with a *look of disapproval* on my face.' Now she began to cry. 'That was the most damaging thing she could have said to me. She put into me all of her own feelings of rejection of me. She made them mine.'

We were quiet for a while. I fought back my own tears, thinking of little Maxine in the photos I had seen of her, with Reuben's eyes. Then she went on.

'Fay was terrified of two things. Cancer and madness. It was phobic. Her own mother, Sarah, had died of pancreatic cancer.'

Susan Sontag wrote of cancer's propensity for cloaking itself in metaphor because of its unclear aetiology: 'cancer fills the role of an illness experienced as a ruthless, secret invasion'.[85] What was the secret invasion of herself that my grandmother feared and had given over to be represented by cancer? I suspected her fear of doctors was a fear of having this unknowable thing in her located and identified. This thing she feared would make her kill Lorrie, and which she felt she had caused. Cancer and madness were one. She could not integrate into herself her own normal bad feelings; they terrified her with their poisonous potential, so mixed up had they become with her illness.

'It seems kind of self-defeating to be scared of cancer and to chain-smoke. And then to be scared of doctors, on top of that,' I pointed out. In the end, Fay died from emphysema and lung cancer in the old-age home. She orchestrated her own real cancerous death. My still-young mother flew back from Australia to live with her at the old-age home for six weeks, where she survived the grimness of her mother's impending death on humour alone, phoning us with stories of octogenarians asking her on dates and the discovery that my grandmother had slept one night in the bathtub, fully clothed and with her walking stick, to avoid a bat that had flown into her room.

I thought back to Fay, ashing her cigarette into the saucer of her teacup in the garden of our house, her wet eyes, her dry mouth. Always a dry mouth. Had she in fact had postnatal psychosis? I knew psychosis in new mothers was considered a far more serious illness in the literature on postnatal depression, because the risk of self-harm or harm to the baby or others is significant. The treatment approach for psychotic illness these days was always medication foremost, specifically antipsychotics, to stop hallucinations or delusions, with psychotherapy in a supportive role to help mother–baby bonding and coping mechanisms. Psychosis generally, in the *Diagnostic and Statistical Manual*, is classified as a disruptive symptom, centrally involving impaired reality testing, of both psychiatric and neurologic conditions. While it certainly causes emotional disturbance, it is approached as a by-product of the organ of the brain more than the mind, perhaps because its manifestations arise via our organs of perception: in hallucinations, in illusions of sensory stimulus. Research into schizophrenia in recent decades has focused on the organ of the brain, too, with promising findings; for example, the discovery in schizophrenic brains of a cellular process that sets off excessive pruning of synaptic connections.

Freud had believed that a psychoanalytic approach to an illness like schizophrenia was impossible, because of the limits delusions and hallucination set in understanding the core therapeutic relationship. He claimed that the narcissistic nature of psychosis, the way it turned the patient's thoughts inward – to the creations of their own ego, rather than to external objects – would prevent the transference developing between the patient and the analyst. But his successor Melanie Klein held that psychosis is fuelled by anxiety, and that a psychotic patient would find relief through the process of analysis if it got to the core of that anxiety.

In the 1950s and '60s, one branch of psychoanalytic thinking did great damage to people with psychosis, specifically schizophrenia (and also to people with autism), with its 'refrigerator mother' theory: that schizophrenia developed in children who were forced to withdraw from the real world in response to cold, unresponsive parents. This was around the time that Fay, who had not officially been diagnosed with psychosis, was coming to terms with her alarming feelings in new motherhood.

Decades later, a diagnosis of postnatal psychosis may have helped her understand that her thoughts of harm were irrational, but back then she probably found herself terrified of the origins of her frightening ideations and too scared to get to the depths of the feelings she now had to deal with in the wake of that experience. A cocktail of too much medication would quiet it all, and would allow her to think of it as only corporeal. Back at an imaginary line between body and mind, and the moral weight of either side of it: the mind, where blame is so often laid, as though suffering is a kind of laziness of soul; the body, where control of the self is lost to the endless replications, divisions and connections made at microscopic levels.

'Did Granny show you love?' I asked her.

'She did. But around the age of four I developed a very serious separation anxiety from her. I was convinced she would not come to get me if I went to a party, or ballet. And it began to get worse. I started school and I had this idea that I might come out at the end of the day and she would not be there to collect me.

'One day, I remember, I was sitting in class looking out the window, and there was a big storm rolling in, as there always was in the afternoons in Johannesburg in summer. I started to panic about what I would do in a storm if Fay was not there waiting in her car. By the time I ran out to where she would usually be, I could not breathe; I was hyperventilating and crying. I was having a panic attack. And she wasn't there. She had parked a little further down the road. But after that, every afternoon I felt the panic come. I just didn't want to go to school. I lost my appetite, and couldn't sleep.'

I wanted to go back in time and put my arms around the little girl Maxine had been. I could see her in my mother still, in her vulnerability. It occurred to me that perhaps my inability to leave her was because I had always sensed the baby in her who had never been held the way she needed to be.

'Fay and your grandpa, Harvey, were worried, but they didn't know what to do. They spoke to the school, and the school psychologist saw me and told them it was separation anxiety. And then for the next few years sometimes I was able to go, and other times I could not go for weeks. It was awful. I lived in fear of Fay's wrath, because sometimes she was kind to me about it and seemed to understand I needed her comfort; other times she was angry with me. Harvey was very angry with me and distanced himself from me completely.

'Then, just before Grade Five, Fay took me and Lorrie on a holiday and I got dangerously sick with food poisoning. They thought I had meningitis, it was so bad. And everything was unsettled at home; we were moving house. But I got better and I felt I could go back to school. I went for the first day, but the panic was overwhelming. I came home and said, *I can never do that again.* The terror was too much.'

Fay's uncertainty about her own capacity to love her child had affected Maxine profoundly – some essential conveying of emotional presence to Maxine that would have, in psychoanalytic terms, made Maxine's freefalling, shapeless anxiety bearable by containing it, giving it borders, turning it into a meaningful concept, was absent. Instead, Fay was in her own terrible state of fear, or possibly disconnect, and Maxine was left in what Wilfred Bion called 'nameless dread', a kind of overwhelming terror that lingers in 'the residue of thoughts and conceptions that have been stripped of their meaning'.[86]

I knew about my mother's school refusal but we hadn't discussed it in years. Once in a while she said something that reminded me what a painful time it had been for her. Around New Year, she would say, 'Oh, I hate all the going-back-to-school ads. They leave me feeling—' and she would clutch at her throat, her heart. Now I understood that sense in me of Maxine freefalling.

I remembered Harvey, Fay's husband and my grandfather, in the way I remembered a storybook character, outlined but not real, in a series of snapshots pastiched from what I saw – always reading the newspaper, bringing meat from delicatessens and fruit home – and what I was told: how, after he was taken captive during World War Two in Tobruk, he had worked on the land near Brindisi, Italy, the place where he began to refuse to eat veal, seeing the calves caged and bloodless. How he lost his language through dementia that was set off by a brain injury when his clothing shop was robbed in the 1980s. His personhood too was irrevocably changed via his body.

'Grandpa Harvey was there, but distant, and as angry as he was with me,' Maxine went on, 'he's the one who got me help. He came home one day with a newspaper clipping from a clinic that said it could help children like me.' The clinic was the Johannesburg Child Guidance Clinic, established in 1944 with a strong psychoanalytic orientation. Children with my mother's kind of problem, school refusal, fell under the clinic's classification of 'neurotic: hysteria, anxiety states, phobias, obsessions'.[87]

'Granny Fay took me there. I'll never forget what I was wearing: a smart lilac suit, buttoned up. And that's when I started seeing Ernest, and it was the first time in my life I had ever felt safe. He told Fay, *There is nothing wrong with Maxine. The problem is with you. You need therapy*. But she never had it; not the kind he offered. She had given up on that. I went there every week for years, but Fay never took me; I had to get a bus on my own. I was only twelve.' The building where she saw Ernest was a four-kilometre drive from home.

My grandmother must have feared Ernest. He would go in with a headlight and scalpel and search for the thing in the ruins, and she would rather the thing stayed hidden.

I'd heard a lot about Ernest from my mother. Seeing him had saved her childhood, by her account, which in turn allowed her to grow up and become a mother. But had my mother also suffered from a postnatal illness? Had whatever had been planted in her as a child – that made her fear her own mother might not be there to collect her after school – remained in her, begun to grow and push outward when she took on the role of mother? Or, if this wasn't about family dynamics, had whatever cerebral misfiring that had caused Fay's postnatal upheaval passed itself on genetically to her?

It was hard to tell, but I'd always thought that in her stories of my birth and my sister's birth there were traces of anguish. Certainly, a focus on how her body failed her. After my sister, her first child, was born, she had come home from the hospital feeling okay, but a week later had begun to bleed massively. Postpartum haemorrhage. I had seen such things in movies. In the year that followed, she had become extremely thirsty, lost a lot of weight, been urinating excessively. Her pancreas wasn't working. It was then she had been diagnosed as a type-1 diabetic. Suddenly, her survival depended on metered doses of insulin, injected into the fat on her abdomen via an ungainly black box, an infusion pump, that she wore at all times. I was conceived while she was finding bodily equilibrium in that new pancreatically deficient self. The story of my entry into the world when told by her has always begun with the incubator they put me in, where they calibrated my blood-sugar levels for three days, which probably gives weight to the level of threat that she felt about her own seemingly failing body and its capacity to house me. But I was fine, a healthy baby. And her body did not fail her in one regard: she breastfed my sister and me with ease and with the fervent adherence of a good La Leche League mother. Breastfeeding, after all, fitted in with psychoanalytic thinking about the primacy of the mother–infant attachment, and if there was one thing my parents were good at it was employing psychoanalytic ideas.

And yet her recollections of my babyhood were speckled with despair, with stories, now told comically, of climbing into my cot out of desperation for sleep in a bid to settle me; of never being able to lay the boundaries between my incessant needs and her survival. The year I was born was the same year my father left her. Attachment, via breastfeeding, to me, and earlier to my sister, was not just the delivery of sustenance to two babies; it was her lifeline. We were her greatest joy, she had told me more times than I could ever count.

'So you're taking your father with you to Holland?' she asked me now. 'You've never asked me to go away with you.'

I wasn't sure what to say. She was right. Maybe I was making up for lost time with Aaron. Or maybe I never asked her because I knew that symbolically I couldn't go anywhere without her.

We pulled up outside the kindergarten. It seemed that, like Lorenz's butterfly, in small and imperceptible ways, and in big and glaring ways, something in the air around each of the mothers before me had come my way.

18

Fay had had postnatal depression and had seen a psychoanalyst, Dr Horwitz, who had medicated her. I wasn't sure how to picture Dr Horwitz in this story. I could imagine a put-upon man with frayed elbow patches reaching for his prescription pad while my grandmother stomped around his office refusing to lie on the couch. But it was possible that he had not treated her as an analyst at all; that he had recognised she was not a candidate for a lengthy self-inquiry, fearful as she was of coming to terms with her guilt, but requiring chemical intervention for the possibly psychotic thoughts she was harbouring.

I had long worried that antidepressants could stall the progress of my therapy; that the altering of emotion through chemicals was anathema to the pursuit of knowing my most hidden self. I worried that the relief those little pills brought me would also stop me getting to the cause of my feelings by masking those feelings. If I wasn't feeling distressed or anxious how could the words I spoke or the way my body moved or the dreams I had offer anything to work with in a therapy that relies on those clues? Where did chemical intervention fit into Adam Phillips's notion that analysis strives to help you *feel realer*? Which of me was the real me? The one who woke with terror in the pit of my guts? Or the one who could enjoy a bowl of porridge once the terror was annihilated? In some sense it was moot. I couldn't get myself to Dr Parkes's rooms each week without those pills.

Beyond my own body, there is a long history to the push

and pull between medication and psychoanalysis, and it gained traction around the time Fay was, possibly, stomping around Dr Horwitz's office.

Over in New York in the 1960s, the psychiatrist and neuroscientist Mortimer Ostow was presenting papers with titles like 'The use of drugs to overcome technical difficulties in psychoanalysis'. Medications, Ostow proposed, could make the patient more receptive to the work by decreasing their defences and increasing the strength of the transference with the therapist. For analysis to at least proceed the patient needs to have insight and be able to examine the interpretations put forward by their analyst, he said, and drugs might put them in a better state of mind to do that. In the same city, the psychoanalyst Thomas Szasz was writing on the ethics of psychoanalysis, where he determined: 'Giving advice and prescribing drugs are frequent causes of imbalance in the analytic relationship [in which] the therapist communicates to the client his readiness to assume some measure of control of the patient's impulses, needs or problems.'[88]

It wasn't until the 1970s, when drugs were beginning to have fewer horrible side effects and biological chemistry was gaining strides, that pharmacology began to dominate mental health care and those Freudian ideas that had been allowed to percolate in psychiatry were dampened. (It was then that the *Diagnostic and Statistical Manual* went into its third edition, the one in which controversy erupted over the deletion of the psychoanalytic concept of *neurosis*.) By the time I was taking my pills and being analysed, there remained stalwart arguments from both the pro-drugs-with-psychoanalysis and anti-drugs-with-psychoanalysis camps. Drugs can confuse the transference and encourage the patient to put up exaggerated defences; drugs can clear symptoms and aid development of trust between patient and analyst; drugs can make psychoanalysis available to people who might not otherwise be able to participate such is their loss of touch with reality, ran some of the arguments.[89] Elyn Saks, the author who detailed her psychoanalytic treatments after her diagnosis of schizophrenia in her memoir *The Centre Cannot Hold*, shows in her story how medication was for her at times essential to address the disordered thinking that came about through her delusions. Then, she could recognise her emotions with clarity and unpack them with her analyst, who 'helped me open a window onto myself, showing me that my psychosis served to protect me from painful thoughts and feelings … knowing that made everything less toxic,' she wrote.[90]

Fay, it turned out, didn't linger long enough in Dr Horwitz's office, let alone on his couch, to test any of this for her future granddaughter. 'She trounced him. She decided she had a chemical disorder and all she needed was the medication. Therapy was useless,' Maxine told me. After that decision, Fay doctor-hopped, going from psychiatrist to psychiatrist. 'She went on anxiolytics; at one point she was on an entirely inappropriate medication, for what they then called manic depression.'

Fay had been a proud homemaker, according to Maxine, but after Dr Horwitz she let things go. I could conjure Fay and Harvey's apartment in Johannesburg so easily still, even though it had been thirty years since I had last set foot in there, on a trip with Joni back to South Africa. I had been eight and Joni ten. We had gone on our own, unaccompanied minors, and stayed half the time at Fay and Harvey's and half the time at the live-in hotel suite where Aaron's mother, Bella, resided. You had to take a trip eight floors up in one of those old birdcage lifts to Fay and Harvey's apartment, and walk along a balcony that looked out toward the city. Their home always smelled of griddle-pan grease from hamburgers, or wurst that Harvey kept wrapped in newspaper in the fridge, and cigarette smoke. Aside from a small collection of Toby Jugs and Royal Doulton figurines on a low antique-wood table, and one ruby-coloured ashtray that seemed precious to my child eyes, they had few belongings and the rest of the apartment was in shabby disarray. The kitchen linoleum peeled off the floor, the bathroom porcelain was cracked. There were burn-holes in the mustard bedspread that covered their spring-worn bed.

I thought then that the apartment was like that because they were getting old and maybe poor too – Harvey was beginning to forget things and neither of them worked anymore – but piecing together what I now know about Fay, there is a hopeless dereliction to it all. She was not attending to the slow decay about them, either because she failed to notice it or because she was numb to it.

Fay's postnatal depression may have had largely physiological origins (the cause of postnatal psychosis, if that's what it was, is unknown but it's thought that hormones, genetics and sleep deprivation play a role) but the effect of it had needed to be regarded emotionally. Instead, by never addressing her profound guilt and fear, Fay's experience had ricocheted down to her own daughters.

I had tried tapering off the antidepressants and failed. Noah had been not quite one and my sleep was still broken. It had been coming up to winter, the sun never quite breaking through. I chose the precipice of nature's retreat, as all the trees were losing their greenness and the lawns were turning to mud, to stop – I could be cruel to myself.

I'd had to do it slowly. At first, I halved the dose every second day, but the brain zaps started, struck me dizzy. I saw the GP: 'You've obviously got a very sensitive metabolism. Try just taking a quarter less every second day.'

It was still too fast. My brain felt as though it moved three seconds after my head. I was like a ten-pin bowling pin on a ship riding wild seas. I'd slowed it down further, shaving bits off the tablets each morning with scissors like a wood sculptor.

And then I was down to nothing, and for a few weeks I'd felt great.

'I'm medication-free!' I'd told Gideon, and we went for dinner to celebrate, where I drank wine and did not feel narcoleptic, as

I had when drinking alcohol on the medication. *I did it*, I told myself. *It was the chemistry of new motherhood; something short-wired in my neurotransmitters. It was hormones!*

I went to Dr Parkes and told him my news. He scribbled in his book. He was going away for a month, and I left the session with a bounce in my step: 'See you in four weeks,' I sang.

Gideon was also going away – two weeks on the other side of Australia for work. 'I'm fine,' I told him. 'It's gone,' I said.

But the pulse of it returned, faint at first, as I watched his taxi pull away from the house. Then, in the middle of the night, when I was woken by Noah calling out. Again, with the sound of a voice calling me for comfort my heart sped up. It came when there was no sound but the burble of the fish-tank filter in the children's bedroom and the shuffle of them falling asleep again, and me waiting in the dark, listening. I tried to breathe slowly.

Gideon was in a different time zone, Dr Parkes was away. The dreams started again, the tsunami ones: I was at a beach and the tide came in rapidly, high. Sometimes Noah or Reuben went under water and I couldn't get to them; sometimes it was I who couldn't get out of the deep water; I clawed at the edge of a concrete wall, tried to lift myself up to safety, but the tug of the ocean was too strong. And the world-end ones: I was standing, looking at the sky; there were two moons. I knew this couldn't be possible; it meant the planets had shifted dangerously. We were hurtling to our deaths. It was the end of humanity. I would not get to say goodbye to my children.

It came in the mornings, even when the dreams were at last fading. I lay in my bed beset by an impermeable doom; not quite thoughts about particular events but a climate of dread in me. The feeling peaked when I thought about taking Reuben to kindergarten and leaving him there. He was happy at kindergarten, but it was a long drive from our house: distance between us seemed to be my struggle again.

The dawn darkness confirmed my sense that beyond the boundaries of my skin, outside the house, in the realm of the living, were all those dangers of separation: the waves that would come, the planetary shifts; an eternal cut-off from safety. I stood at the kitchen counter breathing deeply, willing Gideon to come back. I asked myself how I could get through the day with myself, with the children, with this thrumming heart and exhaustion, with this skittery-rabbit feeling in my throat, my stomach.

During the weeks Gideon was gone I read and read and read to both of them, their bodies nestled into mine. The words stopped my thinking. Dr Seuss, those lengthy tales and sonorous rhythms; poetry – 'The Jabberwocky', in whose nonsense sounds I could unloose my mind. Winnicott believed that the capacity to be alone in the presence of the mother is a fundamental step in the psychological development of the child. The child who can be in the presence of someone but be so absorbed in their internal space that they are not impinged upon by the demands of the other person. Reading to the children made me feel I was protecting them from my messy internal space; they were with me but not with my anxiety, which betrayed me in my body in certain ways: the speed with which I did things, the way I was always moving my head from shoulder to shoulder to relieve the tension of those muscles. Often I thought of Maxine, tried to remember her reading with me or playing with me as a small child, wondered if she too had closed her eyes as she turned a page, dragged down by the swamp of exhaustion anxiety brought, let her face go slack, or even cried quietly while Joni and I faced away from her.

In reading there was hope for us all: 'the child confronts the idea of terror through story and confronts it in the presence of a containing mind which offers hope that thoughts can become thinkable', writes the academic Daniel Brass, who draws from Bion's ideas about how a mother offers an infant a way to cope with primitive feelings by providing words that turn those frightening sensations of experience into thought.[91] I hoped that whatever amorphous terror I brought to the children through the signals of my own despair might be more manageable for them in the form of the Jabberwock, 'with eyes of flame ... whiffling through the tulgey wood', whom we could shut away in his pages at the end of the poem.

I had had a clear thought one morning: *I am finding living harder than I remember it ought to be.* I dropped a small white pill onto my tongue and started again.

And then Gideon had returned, and Dr Parkes had come back, and once again it was impossible to know what had caused what in me.

The data on the effectiveness of medication for postnatal depression was, like my own way of understanding my narrative, speckled with inconclusiveness. The most recent high-quality review of antidepressants for PND concluded that current evidence across all studies is of a very low quality. Reasons for this were a risk of bias in the included studies (in particular, high proportions of participants dropping out) and the exclusion of women with long-lasting or severe depression, or both. The review also concluded that current research is limited by the lack of data on long-term follow-up (including on the safety of breastfeeding or child outcomes), and that overall larger studies need to be done.[92]

While the review did conclude that women with postnatal depression who were given selective serotonin reuptake inhibitors (SSRIs, the sort of antidepressant I was on) were more likely to improve or recover than those given a placebo, there was not enough evidence across the data available to answer whether antidepressants work better than other treatments. Are antidepressants or psychosocial/psychological treatments more effective, and for whom? Are some antidepressants more effective or better tolerated than others? The papers also did not seem to differentiate between the notion of anxiety and the notion of depression in a woman experiencing PND, which perhaps reflected the way the *DSM* categorised anxiety as part of a broader 'peripartum major depressive episode'.

Lacking any definitive answers, the review recommended that treatment decisions for women with PND use evidence from other sources, such as trials in general adult populations. It also recommended that future studies include women with severe postnatal depression, and that there be a long-term follow-up on psychiatric symptoms and quality of life in mothers who have been treated for postnatal depression.

Another review, conducted around the same time, was similarly unable to come to conclusions about the effectiveness of antidepressants for PND – data is too limited, sample sizes are too small, populations being studied are too diverse, attrition rates are too high – but was more emphatic in its assessment of the current state of research: 'Given that postpartum depression is a major public health problem, it is surprising that the controlled data consist of only 6 randomized trials including 3 placebo-controlled studies.'[93]

In Australia alone, the prevalence of PND – as well as the economic burden it brings, both indirectly through productivity loss and directly through health-care costs – makes the weakness of the data surprising. The peak body for perinatal anxiety and depression support, PANDA, says that anxiety or depression during pregnancy and up to one year after birth affects around 100,000 families annually. That's not an insignificant amount, on a par with the number of individuals per year who develop diabetes in Australia.[94] The economic effect is notable: the money spent on health services related to PND in 2012, according to a study commissioned for PANDA, amounted to around $78 million, with productivity losses associated with PND just over $310 million (a number that includes productivity losses for fathers affected by their own or their partner's PND).[95]

The clinical practice guidelines for effective mental health care in the perinatal period, which gives evidence-based recommendations for health professionals, offered me no more clarification on my personal conundrum than the reviews had.[96] It stated that the body of evidence for psychodynamic therapy for women diagnosed with mild to moderate depression in the postnatal period was weak, and while it could be recommended as a treatment it must be 'applied with caution'.

As for medication, the guidelines concluded there was insufficient evidence from studies in antenatal or postnatal populations regarding the efficacy of antidepressant medication, and insufficient evidence from studies in antenatal or postnatal populations regarding the pharmacological treatment of anxiety disorders.

Insufficient evidence. Insufficient evidence. I was coming up against dead ends wherever I turned.

In 2017, the clinical practice guidelines were updated. New data showed fewer than 20 per cent of cases of perinatal mental health conditions come to the attention of health-care practitioners. A recommendation was made that every woman be screened at multiple points during pregnancy and postnatally using a standard questionnaire to allow for early intervention.

Also, a 'consensus-based recommendation' (one formulated in the absence of quality evidence) had been made about psychological intervention for women with moderate to severe anxiety and depressive disorders. It suggested that 'psychological intervention is a useful adjunct, usually once medications have become effective', but gave no specific advice on psychodynamic or psychoanalytic therapy. The review heartily recommended cognitive behavioural therapy or interpersonal therapy (a brief form of structured therapy that focuses on a person's relationships and life events), each of which has a clear-cut evidence base, but therapy that involved the unconscious mind was not addressed.

The new recommendations also made evidence-based recommendations for the use of SSRIs as first-line treatment for moderate to severe depression and/or anxiety in pregnant and postnatal women, and a consensus-based recommendation of short-term benzodiazepine use while waiting for SSRI or tricyclic antidepressants to take effect for women with moderate to severe perinatal anxiety.[97]

So the evidence base for pharmacological treatments for perinatal depression was gaining strength, but a bigger question hovered over an area that could not be separated out from this: the mechanism of antidepressants generally. No one knows how they work or, arguably, whether they work at all.

Until the late 1980s, depression had been treated with tricyclic antidepressants (named after their chemical structure), which the psychiatrist Roland Kuhn had discovered quite by accident in Switzerland in the 1950s.

Kuhn had been using a medication on schizophrenic patients that he noticed seemed to help their depression. The drug affected two brain chemicals that communicate information between nerve cells (which are called neurotransmitters) to control mood and pain: dopamine and norepinephrine. By 1957, he had conducted enough studies on his depressed patients to publish a paper on what was then the first medication targeting mood disorders: imipramine. It was something of a wonder, a chemical that could lift mood, but it also caused serious side effects: huge weight gain, sluggishness. And it had an overdose risk. Nevertheless, along with tranquillisers (mainly the kind known as anxiolytics, which slow down signals between our brain cells and are highly dependence-producing), tricyclics remained the first line of pharmacological treatment for depression and anxiety for the next thirty years.

Toward the end of the 1980s, researchers zeroed in on a different line of medication that worked on a neurotransmitter called serotonin. Serotonin regulates the passing of messages between nerve cells in a range of physiological functions to do with feeding, aggression and sleep, and when targeted it does not cause the side effects of the tricyclic pills.

The new medications were called selective serotonin reuptake inhibitors. Their therapeutic effect supposedly lies in increasing the levels of serotonin in the brain's synapses. The problem is there has never been evidence to show that serotonin needs tweaking in patients with depression or anxiety, nor has there been evidence to show whether SSRIs in fact do increase serotonin levels.

Animal studies have cast significant doubt on whether the serotonin neuronal system is the key to depression. One study even showed that mice that have been genetically manipulated so that their serotonin pathways are disrupted do not show depressed behaviours.[98] The rodent version of depressed behaviours includes freezing in a situation of stress rather than trying to escape (controversially, this is shown through a tail-suspension test, during which the mouse is hung by its tail around ten centimetres from the ground, or a swim test in which the mouse is dropped into water and left to swim with no route to exit the water). It also includes anhedonia, or indifference to reward (observed by offering the mouse plain water or sucrose-infused water).

That same study also showed that, while SSRIs might alter our levels of depression, it might not be for the reasons we have supposed. Both mice with normal serotonin pathways and those with disrupted pathways had the same response to the SSRIs: both moved more in the stress situations than they did without the SSRIs. Perhaps some other mechanism entirely is at work.

Serotonin may well be part of the picture but it's probably not the whole picture. According to professor of psychiatry David Healy, 'Just as with … other neurotransmitters, we can expect it to vary among individuals and expect some correlation with temperament and personality.'

In a 2015 editorial in the *British Medical Journal*, Healy concluded that the rise of SSRIs is an example of a plausible but mythical account of biology being marketed in the face of clear clinical trial evidence to the contrary. A case of a good narrative getting in the way of facts. For this, he blames the vast terrain of modern neuroscience: 'the emerging sciences of the brain offer enormous scope to deploy any amount of neurobabble'.

Healy's words imply a conspiracy if taken at face value – one that would implicate layers of doctors, pharmacists, researchers. But the problem is likely less sinister and more to do with number-crunching, and the weight given to journal-published data. Antidepressant research outcomes are liable, as with all clinical trial research, to be skewed by what is known as publication bias: the selection of positive outcomes for journal publication. In America, for example, the US Food and Drug Administration (FDA) ensures the visibility of all drug trials and makes them accessible for review, but not all the negative trials make it as published articles in the journals that are read by doctors and prescribers. The positive outcomes usually outweigh the negative ones in the publication stakes.

In 2008, a group of researchers headed by psychiatry researcher Erick H Turner looked at reviews from the FDA for a total of 74 studies of a range of antidepressants involving 12,564 patients. They then conducted a literature review to see which outcomes had been reported in journals, and found that studies the FDA viewed as having negative or questionable results were either never published in journals or were published with a positive spin. The result of this skewing effect is that, according to the published literature, it looks like 94 per cent of the trials were positive, where the FDA analysis showed only 51 per cent to be positive.[99] There is a push to rectify this bias by providing platforms for clinical trial data to be registered worldwide for public access (for example, the register Alltrials.net) but it will take some time for this data to become cumulatively useful.

The murkiness of mood-disorder pharmacology research outcomes has spawned a series of intellectual spars among psychiatrists – and a number of *New York Times* bestsellers. Peter D Kramer's 1993 book *Listening to Prozac* argued for the person-changing capabilities of SSRIs, but within a decade the mice were being hung and the doubt was creeping in and Kramer was being refuted by others, most notably Irving Kirsch, whose 2008 meta-analysis of published and unpublished trials on SSRIs concluded that they only have an effect on severe depression, as in cases of milder depression the effect they have is no better than a placebo.[100] What's more, he hypothesised, the response seen in the more severe cases of depression was not an indication of the drug actually working. Instead, what was happening was that the higher doses of medication being given to those with more severe cases were resulting in stronger side effects, making those participants aware they were on the drugs, not the placebo, and this awareness was causing a kind of paradoxical, ramped-up placebo effect.

Kirsch went on to write a book, *The Emperor's New Drugs: exploding the antidepressant myth*, that claimed previous assertions of the efficacy of SSRIs were the result of cherry-picking and faulty consensus in studies. Kramer followed up in 2016 with *Ordinarily Well: the case for antidepressants*, in which he made a convincing argument that the problem with antidepressant research lies not in the evidence about whether SSRIs work (they do for some, though he acknowledges that how they work is unclear) but in the way pharmacological studies had abandoned the kind of subjectivity and personal observation that was essential to early scientific knowledge about depression treatment.

In 2017, yet another paper came out, this time refuting Kirsch's placebo-effect conclusions.[101] That study conducted an analysis of trial studies for two SSRIs, and found a clinically significant improvement in the mood of patients given SSRIs compared with those given placebos, regardless of whether the SSRI caused them to experience side effects: 'our results indirectly support the notion that the two drugs under study do display genuine antidepressant effects caused by their pharmacodynamic properties'. In other words, the side-effect hypothesis was debunked.

Kirsch remained sceptical. He responded to the paper by criticising its methodology, and arguing that the difference between the assessments of the patients' depressed moods on placebos and on SSRIs (registered on a measure called the Hamilton Depression Rating Scale) was so minuscule as to have no clinical meaning, and that other factors may have caused the small improvement: 'at least part of this tiny difference between drug and placebo may actually be due to something not related to side effects ... we don't have enough data right now to really know for sure'.[102]

Then, in 2018, a robust study – the biggest analysis of published and unpublished antidepressant-outcome research to date – concluded that twenty-one antidepressant medications (including SSRIs, the older tricyclic antidepressants, and the more recently developed SNRIs that affect serotonin and noradrenaline transmitters, which get cells ready for action) were more effective than a placebo for adults suffering a major depressive disorder.[103]

The clinically significant mood improvement attributed to SSRIs in the 2017 study, and this more recent and wider-ranging 2018 study, offer some assurance for a pharmaceutical approach to depression. But since there is yet to be evidence of any disorder of serotonin function among people with psychiatric diagnoses, or clear evidence of a failure of other specific neurotransmitters among them, do these results bring us any closer to knowing what causes this kind of mental suffering? The hypothesis that these medications are fixing neurotransmitter problems 'is all an inference from the effect of the drugs', claim sociologist Hillary Rose and neuroscientist Steven Rose in their examination of the bioscience industry *Genes, Cells and Brains: the Promethean promises of the new biology*.[104] In fact, they may be doing something else entirely, or nothing at all.

But so what? Who cares, if they work, right? David Healy says the problem with focusing on a neurotransmitter that we can only infer is responsible for depression, like serotonin, is that it distracts from research into 'established biological disturbances' linked to depression. For example, we could be focusing on raised cortisol, which is a hormone released during stress, and also on the role of the neurotransmitter glutamate, which raises excitability in the nervous system. Healy blames drug companies for the 'myth' that serotonin is the key to depression and anxiety. He claims they 'marketed SSRIs for depression, even though they were weaker than older tricyclic antidepressants, and sold the idea that depression was the deeper illness behind the superficial manifestations of anxiety'.[105] We may be looking at the deer in the foreground while the tiger lurks behind.

Some argue the research focus on anxiolytics, which help reduce anxiety, may likewise be misplaced. Aside from SSRIs, the main chemical treatment for anxiety has been benzodiazepines, an anxiolytic that came on to the market in the 1960s after chemist Leo Sternbach discovered its sedative, anticonvulsant and muscle-relaxing properties in animal studies.

Neuroscientist Joseph LeDoux summarises the criticisms of anxiolytic drug research in his book *Anxious: the modern mind in the age of anxiety*. Many of his points come back to problems that arise in animal subjects. He says that anxiety studies typically only assess the temporary state created by a manufactured threat (state anxiety) in animals, and that the kind of anxiety experienced by humans looking for a pharmacological solution is a different kind of thing: a chronic condition (trait anxiety). Further, subject selection in animal studies (where rats are randomly chosen from a colony without knowledge of whether they have chronic anxiety conditions equivalent to a human with trait anxiety) means the research is not particularly helpful in relation to a pathological state of anxiety in humans. He also points out that animal studies usually involve single-drug administration, when many psychiatric drugs take weeks to show an effect in humans. Benzodiazepines will show an effect on humans after one dose, but other anxiolytics may not, and this methodology excludes discovering potential new treatments in that category.

Finally, one of his most interesting criticisms is that animal models usually focus on males, but in human populations women are far more likely than men to develop anxiety disorders.[106] No wonder the pharmacology of perinatal depression is understudied. There's probably a wealth of anxious rat mothers out there doing circles of their backyard trying to get their baby rats to sleep, hoping to be selected for drug trials.

Look at this confident claim from a 2011 paper on how images produced using radiation technology (fMRIs) can pinpoint the physiological origins of anxiety disorder: 'It is now well established that gabaergic, noradrenergic and serotonergic systems play a critical role in … anxiety disorders, abnormalities in these systems being related to structural and functional alterations in specific brain areas … as repeatedly shown by neuroimaging studies.'[107]

Then read what Rose and Rose have to say about fMRIs: 'The dramatic false-colour images that grace the journal articles and media reports of fMRI studies are the result of extensive mathematical transformations of the raw observations of blood flow … at best they are mere cartography – providing maps but no explanations of causative mechanisms.'[108]

The more you wade into the studies and criticisms and op-eds on pharmacological treatments, the deeper you get into disputes like this: corrections and statements of relativism about what should be considered good evidence that lead to little clarity for the person deciding whether or not to pop a little white pill onto their tongue in the dark of a winter bathroom that seems to be closing in around them.

19

The trip to Holland was fast approaching. I had managed to schedule an interview with Mark Solms, who would be the keynote speaker, and I was clutching at any free time between kindergarten drop-off and cleaning out food containers and changing nappies and organising passports to read as much as I could on psychoanalysis and neuropsychoanalysis before the conference.

I went to Aaron and Paul's house to scour through some boxes in their garage in which Aaron had suggested I might find some reading material. They had turned the garage into a family shrine: photos of Joni's and my weddings, baby and kindergarten shots of the grandchildren all framed, hung on the unfinished brickwork around their car.

In one box I found Aaron's meandros collection. Meandros is the Greek letter that symbolises both wandering and wondering. He had a meandros ring, and plate, and business cards. He was thrilled and surprised to discover, long after he began the collection, that the meandros was being used as the logo for the Freud Museum in London. My father loves this kind of coincidence; nothing we do is trivial, arbitrary or haphazard, Freud said of mental life. I did not take the meandros paraphernalia; instead, I took two ceramic horses that I found in newspaper at the bottom of the box. I remembered them sitting on a table in his consulting rooms when I was a child. I was always quick to take something of Aaron's to keep.

Going through my father's discarded books was a luxury for me. I had so rarely had access to his belongings. In my mother's house, I had an intimacy with the objects that surrounded her, with the books that lined her shelves. Nadine Gordimer, Athol Fugard, Agatha Christie, and she had the Freud set too, Winnicott, Klein – I knew the authors' names in the way that I had learned by rote strange words that had no meaning to me yet, like the sign on the elevators around Johannesburg that I could say but not translate from Afrikaans: *In geval van vuur moenie die hysers gebruik nie* (*In case of fire do not use lifts*, I later found out). The feel of those books, the dust jackets, the paperbacks. I'd test the bottle of Dior on her armoire, use the Palmolive moisturiser on her bedside table, take from the half-empty boiled sweet packet beside it in case of midnight sugar lows. In each maternal house of my childhood there were expanses of time to be in the presence of its belongings – later, when my mother was married to my stepfather, my knowledge of the house's belongings was hemmed in, confined to the rooms not haunted by my stepfather's late wife.

I was never in my father's house long enough for that kind of acquaintance with his things. He and Paul had no doubt missed that contact with Joni and me too – they had surprised us on one visit back to see them with new, beautifully decorated rooms for each of us, with patchwork linen and white wrought-iron bed frames. That they kept those rooms, two extra spaces in their homes for the children who only visited them a handful of times a year, showed me how much they wanted our presence.

I had gotten to know my father's professional reading material, because there was often time, on my visits back to Perth, to be whiled away in his consulting rooms while he caught up on paperwork – it was on those shelves that I became familiar with Freud and the other analysts. But there was a familiarity with the objects he lived with that I lacked, and this came not only from the distance between our living quarters but from how I turned away from seeing the things that my father did not feel needed hiding. Much as I had felt when he had first told me he was gay, it was not his sexual orientation that I wanted to shield myself from but his openness of sexual expression. I was shy about anything to do with sex, squeamish even. Later, as an adult, when I was coming to see how much I struggled to separate from Maxine, it dawned on me that this was an expression of wanting to stay a child. A child who does not know about sex does not need to enter the adult world and leave the safety of their mother.

So in my father's house I did not look. Once I was an older child, and he and Paul no longer hid their relationship from Joni and me, I avoided their room, rarely venturing past the door. Looking closely, in my father's house, threatened exposure to things I still found too confronting. I had already encountered the small replica statue of David, with his glaring male genitalia, upon the bathroom counter. There was the Marquis de Sade etching, with its muted tones, somehow illicit in conjuring more of shadow than light. Once in a while I would realise a paperback I had lifted from the bookshelf bore a homoerotic storyline, naked male buttocks adorning its front. Instead of feeling an invitation to sexual freedom in the discovery of these items, I took a kind of shame upon myself for finding them, as though it was I who had come upon something I should not have found. It was safer to feel this way about my father than to feel he had been so insensitive to my childhood feelings that he had not thought to temper his own inherent exhibitionism to allow me to confront sexuality in the quiet way I needed to.

Nor had my father gotten to know me through my belongings. I thought of the way that every day I carefully shelved and reordered all of the books, toys and ornaments that Reuben and Noah had. I knew their toy collection in detail: the missing head on Hulk, the button that no longer worked on the motorised tractor. I knew in the dark at midnight when I went in to soothe Reuben to find his moon torch exactly between the gold plastic medal he was coveting and the stone he had found in the garden and painted yellow. My father could not have known those things about my childhood rooms.

That day, in their garage, with unfettered access to my father's personal books, I felt acutely the distance that existed between us in knowing each other, and the ways I had avoided knowing him. I left with a copy of the old Wulf Sachs book Maxine had told me she had read as a teenager – the one that had gotten her hooked on Freud. She had told me she'd borrowed the book from the library before she knew my father. But now I wondered if Aaron had lent it to her once they met. Or it was possible they each had come across their own copies? The true course of events in any life is barely traceable once human memory enters the picture.

If you follow the meandros pattern on the border of a Greek urn you realise its central aesthetic quality is the way it provides infinitesimal possible visual routes.

After I had visited the Buddhist therapist and considered going onto medication, when Reuben was six months old, back at my house in Melbourne I had phoned him to ask if they could send me a note letting me know what kind of medication I had been on in the years I had seen him. I thought it would be helpful to know what had worked for me in the past. Through some misjudgement or oversight, the receptionist sent me photocopies of my entire therapeutic history as recorded by the Buddhist therapist. I flicked through it with horror, sensing that if I read it I would find out a terrifying truth about myself. It felt dangerous, a Rosetta stone. I shoved it back in its big yellow envelope, and caught the last page as it missed and fluttered to the floor. *Has a disproportionate ideation of her father, whom she sees as perfect and all good*, it said, in the Buddhist's balanced scrawl.

I recoiled, felt shame wash over me. It was one thing to adore your father when you were a child. Freud's whole theory of infantile sexuality rested on the child's passionate love for their parent of the opposite sex. But had I, even as an adult, been unable to see fault in my father? I found it hard to view him negatively, when I thought about it, even despite his obvious grand infraction of leaving our household, or his smaller faults of insensitivity to my prudishness. It had been easy to feel adulation for him as I was growing up in the turmoil of my mother and stepfather's household. Then, I would fly back to Perth with Joni and spend calm, luxurious leisure time in his house in Perth with Paul, where there was always a festive air, food being prepared, beach outings and picnics and movies at open air cinemas. Twenty-five years later, when the awful marriage-equality vote was being cast in Australia, I wished I could teleport the politicians claiming same-sex marriage would harm children back into my childhood, where the model I had of a loving, peaceful home was in Aaron and Paul's house.

Then, my father would take Joni and me to the video store, and give us free rein in the films we chose. I honed a sense of the ridiculous on those holidays, watching Steve Martin and Mel Brooks movies. He brought me tea in the morning when I woke, he played Trivial Pursuit with us, took us to museums and the Fremantle markets, waited with endless patience while I trawled soap and stationery and gemstone aisles looking to spend the allowance he had given me. Time with Aaron was holiday time. The marital dysfunction of my maternal household aside, it also stood in vast contrast to the pressured domestic necessities of home life: my endless battles with my mother over the unloading of the dishwasher, the putting away of washing. With my father and Paul in Perth, the whole holiday was organised around Joni's and my entertainment. Aaron took leave from work, booked bike tours and day trips. I had my father completely then.

And he was unfailingly temperate. He never raised his voice at me. It had become family folklore that the one and only time he had gotten openly angry was when he'd lost his patience with Joni one afternoon after she left one of her shoes at the public swimming pool and we'd had to pile back into the car to get it.

I had never fought with my father. My mother and I, on the other hand, had a pattern of devastating, explosive arguments that left us both disoriented. They would begin with some relatively banal act on my part – putting a mug on the wooden table without a coaster, or opening the blinds too roughly. She lived in fear of my stepfather's fuse, and she relentlessly exerted control over my sister and me as proxies for the house that she felt did not belong to her, with its grand antiques procured by my stepfather and his previous wife, who had died young and whose beatified portrait hung above my stepfather's desk. Countless times I had been so unhinged with rage at Maxine that I had run away from our house into the park down the road, where I had wept and repeatedly punched my hand into the soft part of my arm. I wanted a bruise to appear as a physical marker of the inexplicable opposition we posed to each other.

But what had happened to my anger at Aaron for leaving us? Was the Buddhist therapist right? Perhaps I had buried and replaced it with a kind of idolatry: safer to worship than to reject a father who has trailed out far, to the edges of disappearing, for a new life. While I knew my mother's emotional life intimately, I knew very little about my father's inner world. It was possible I had skirted around asking him direct questions for fear of what he might tell me.

'Is your sister's birthday the ninth or the tenth of March?' he asked me once. I was stunned that he couldn't remember such a momentous date. My children's birthdates were seared in my memory like the spelling of my own name. 'Well, it's just that your mother and I got married on the tenth, so I get them muddled up.' I was flummoxed. I had never thought to wonder when they had gotten married. That there was a date to commemorate it, and that my father still held onto it, was as startling to me as my discovery had been, aged four, that the moon did not change shape but was merely in shadow from time to time.

It had only been recently that I first saw photos of their

wedding, in an album I unpacked for my mother when she arrived to live near me in Melbourne. I had turned the pages aghast, feeling I had stumbled upon something deliberately lost. Because of the silence around it, I had obliterated the notion of the event from my imagination altogether. There were no artefacts remaining from it either: no wedding dress kept in tissue paper, cards of congratulations, ring. I had no idea what they had done with their wedding rings. I had carefully curated the evidence of their unity from the story of my self, in case it should reveal itself to be a sham. Reconstructing too elaborately the celebration of their unity might lead me into my father's head, where I might find him admiring his groomsmen or thinking about sneaking off to have an affair with the young male dish-hand in the hotel scullery while my mother reapplied her lipstick in the marital suite.

There was a story my father told me as an adult about how he almost drowned shortly after my mother and he married. They were on a beach holiday, and he was in the water with a friend when they got caught in a rip. They were saved by a teenager who saw them struggling. 'We nearly died,' he told me. In my mind that story got conflated somehow with my parents' wedding, so that I had once started telling a friend how my father went swimming after his wedding and nearly drowned, but quickly realised the impossibility of this: they had married in landlocked Johannesburg. I saw then how deeply my parents' union was tied up with a sense in me that I almost never existed.

I had never asked Aaron how much he knew about himself when he married my mother. I felt the answer might somehow undo me; if he had known already he was gay, known he was going to leave us, I might have been created with regret, or ambivalence, or, worse, a hope that I never fulfilled. Better to keep him in a frieze of obliviousness, blindsided.

20

Maxine and I met once a week at a cafe around the corner from both our houses, in an outdated shopping plaza that served more as a gathering point for elderly men than as a business. The men occupied two separate camps according to ethnicity: the Italians played cards at one cafe and the Greeks played backgammon at another. At a third cafe, run by an Italian woman that my mother had befriended, we would sit among the jars of passata and windows of cannoli and drink our coffees. My mother greeted almost every customer who came in, explaining to me, *sotto voce*, as they passed, their story: *She's married to the owner of that big burger chain that was sued. Open marriage. That guy – he used to be everyone's gardener. Nice man.*

My mother was interested in other people. She never forgot a face. 'Your mother has an eidetic memory,' my father said often. I shared her penchant for the lurid, odd, criminal. In all people, we recognised, was the capacity for both the utterly ordinary and the curiously dark. We knew it in ourselves. My quest to trace what had happened to me as a new mother – grave and in some ways as humiliating as I found it – was lit by a kind of excitement too; I was a puzzle as available to forensic dissection as a murderer on *Law & Order*. And often my conversations with my mother were a kind of root-cause analysis. Today I was cross-examining her. Did we have a family history of any kind that related to my emotional experiences?

'Your grandmother Fay called it a sickness. She said, *It's a sickness and it's in the family*,' Maxine told me. 'Fay developed her own psychiatric history, claiming depression was in the family. *Endogenous depression*. She'd read it somewhere. She read extensively, self-diagnosed. She had medical misbeliefs. Thank god she was never computer literate.'

Fay had adored her own mother, Sarah. Doted on her. Had seen her as a beautiful, gentle bird in need of protection. 'But what would she need protection from?' I asked.

'Her husband was a terrible womaniser,' my mother offered. 'Actually, she wasn't a gentle bird, either. She was passive aggressive. Seething quietly with anger. *Farribledick*.' This was a Yiddish word; it connoted a person beset by minor annoyances with others. 'But, you know, that was the generation. Sarah didn't speak to her own mother for years over some minor infraction.' The *generation* my mother was referring to were the late-nineteenth-century Jewish immigrants who came to South Africa from small towns in pre-Holocaust Eastern Europe, or *shtetls*. Towns so tiny and often intrinsically insular from a self-protection against pervasive anti-Semitism that neighbourly nitpicking and in-fighting were a veritable local sport.

'And Granny Fay's sister?' I remembered my great-aunt Maya clearly. She always wore red lipstick and would kiss me full on my lips in greeting. There was always drama between Fay and Maya. I could never follow what had happened.

'Yes, Maya. But there was also Fay's brother George.' I had forgotten about George and recalled immediately that his story was somehow tragic; my ability to erase him from memory so easily signalled to me his story must have frightened me deeply.

'God, George! Of course! What happened to him again?'

The story of George spooled from her as all her stories did, vivid as film. George was the youngest, and the family revered him. He was extremely good-looking and engaging, university educated, political. 'Everybody hated everybody in the family, but they loved George,' my mother said. My mother told me that in the mid 1950s, when she was three, George fell in love with a beautiful young woman, Brenda, from Cape Town. But the fairytale quickly took on a hint of foreboding. 'Someone went to Granny Sarah and told her that Brenda had been in a mental institution and was schizophrenic.' The family promptly flew into an insulted rage at the bearer of this news, feeling the gossiper was being malicious. But they worried, too. What if it were true?

George and Brenda, who I imagine felt keenly the cloistering watchfulness of the family, left to live in London and contacted the family back in Johannesburg less often than my great-granny Sarah would have liked. But news got back that they were trying to have a baby, and after a long enough time to cast an anxious pall on their fertility, Brenda fell pregnant. Their little girl was born and named Georgina, news of which once again ignited the family's worry – in Jewish custom it was bad luck to name a baby after a living family member.

Despite the judgement of the family falling on them, within weeks of the baby's birth they brought her back to Johannesburg. My mother remembered their arrival. 'It was … shocking. Georgina had severe brain damage.' George and Brenda soon left for Cape Town, and returned without Georgina, whom they gave over to an institution.

'I remember Brenda sitting in our lounge room. She never spoke, just cried.' My mother was in the midst of her school refusal at this point. Witnessing the parental abandonment of Georgina can't have impacted her lightly.

Things fell apart for George and Brenda. They returned to London where reports reached the South African family that Brenda was psychotic and had been hospitalised. The marriage ended. George was heartbroken, and his family blamed Brenda. Likely recoiling from this final blow of their disapproval in his choice of partner, George withdrew from his family, having minimal contact with them even when his mother, Granny Sarah, died in 1968.

Word somehow got back to Johannesburg that Brenda had died of breast cancer, and that George had remarried, but then – nothing.

'Until 1973,' my mother said. 'I just remember the phone ringing and my mother answering it and screaming *My baby brother, my baby brother!*'

George had committed suicide. He swallowed cyanide.

What was this *sickness in the family* my grandmother had talked about? Could my postnatal experience be reduced to biological terms, to nature: an aberration in my DNA? Or was it that over the generations patterns of relating, emotional dynamics, had sent generalised anxiety or depression down the line like dominoes? Studies of babies and then the adults they become have shown that those early infant responses to separation influence our adult emotional partnerships.[109] It seemed likely they would also influence our parental attachments. Peter Fonagy had shown, in his studies, that a mother's attachment to her parents directly shaped her neurochemistry, and therefore her chemical responses to her own baby. My mother feared her mother wouldn't be there; my mother's mothering was fraught with this fear, with attempts to keep me close, perhaps made worse by my father leaving; I in turn embodied a fear of being separated from her, and when I had my own children I fell into a panic both because of the separation, bodily, from them that birth required, and the separation, emotionally, from my mother, that becoming a mother myself required.

One 2011 study claims that postnatal depression is transmitted across generations: 'women whose mothers had suffered from postnatal depression had an average score for postpartum depression symptoms that was significantly higher than women whose mothers did not report this. Likewise, women with a score indicating symptoms of postpartum depression more often had mothers who were also more likely to report having suffered from postpartum depression during their life.'

The study looked at a series of questionnaires completed by sixty-five postpartum women and their mothers, including the Edinburgh Postnatal Depression Scale for the new mothers and the Bromley Postnatal Depression Scale for their mothers, which is a tool for retrospective diagnosis of postnatal depression; two surveys intended to measure the quality of their mother–daughter relationship and quality of attachment. The study itself acknowledges the results must be read cautiously both for the study's low participant rate and its reliance on retrospective recall, which can result in an overvaluation of symptoms and their length, but it suggests our mothers' stories cannot be overlooked in our own experience of mothering.[110]

Psychoanalyst Alice Miller had a psychological theory about how emotional trauma might be passed down a family line. She said that in order to grow into emotionally healthy adults we need an experience of early childhood in which we are regarded and respected for who we are. If we are not treated this way, and instead our parents forgo our actual feelings to fulfill their emotional needs, we develop a false self and move to our unconscious minds those experiences of being treated inauthentically. It is those traumas we have hidden away, and that false self, which never truly feels in a healthy way, that causes our adult mental suffering. Unless we can decipher, in therapy, these intense adult emotions and their rudimentary connections with our original childhood experiences, we will continue to carry them around with us as adults. And, what's more, we will spend our adult lives in a state of searching for what caused the trauma – what our parents did not give us emotionally – inflicting this same trauma on our children, for, 'the most efficacious objects for substitute gratification are the parent's *own children*'.[111]

Miller, a Polish Jew who had survived the Holocaust after escaping the Piotorkow ghetto but who'd had to suppress her own hatred for her mother on account of the bigger external-world threat of the Nazis, was in the end her own best evidence for this theory. After her death, her son, Martin, published a book in which he detailed the abuse and emotional neglect he suffered as a child at the hands of the great Alice Miller. 'Alice Miller did the very opposite of what she wrote – but I do not say that what she wrote is wrong. If I hadn't been familiar with her theory, I would be dead today: My mother's theory helped me survive,' Martin has said. The tragedy of a mother who spent her lifetime penning a solution to free her son from her own tyranny.[112]

Alice Miller used a language of biology to talk about the transmission of emotional dysfunction, which she referred to as 'the knowledge stored inside our bodies', the child's repressed emotions staying 'in her cells, stored up as information that can be triggered by a later event'.[113] Was this mere metaphor for a psychoanalytic idea of the way the unconscious mind bids us to act based on our own hidden-away traumas, or was it prescience about matters that the science of genetics would only catch up to decades later?

The science on the genetics of psychological traits is complicated. First, there is the problem that humans experience mental or emotional disturbances in such varying ways, so psychiatric genetic studies need vast numbers of participants to increase the likelihood of clear genomic patterns being pinpointed. Second, as we now know through the emerging field of epigenetics – the study of the material in our genes that causes them to express themselves or remain dormant – genes switch on and off (to borrow the image oft used to convey their functioning) depending on interaction with other genetic material and environmental factors.

This idea that an aspect of a person has been inherited genetically but requires other factors to manifest becomes clearer if we look at a species that is genetically uniform but can have 'castes' or different roles and correspondingly different physiological features. In an ant colony, for example, you might have a soldier ant with a broad head and strong mandibles, and you might have a drone with a small head and tiny mandibles. Studies by a team at the University of Pennsylvania and New York University have discovered that, although genetically all ants in the colony are the same, the ants' genes are activated differently: there is a biochemical system at work that affects the switching on and off of their genes, and synthetic chemicals administered to the brains of young ants will alter the ants' neuronal activity and cause them to behave like ants from a different caste.[114] As the biological scientist Siddhartha Mukherjee put it in the *New Yorker*: 'All of the ants' possible selves are inscribed in its genome. Epigenetic signals conceal some of these selves and reveal others … the ant chooses a life between its genes and its epigenes, inhabiting one self among its incipient selves.'[115]

The field of epigenetics says that we might inherit our parents' genes, but that our own life factors might decide whether or not a particular gene is activated. For postnatal anxiety, or perinatal depression, as the *DSM-5* defined my experience, interpreting the research data on genetics might therefore ask not only *Can I understand what happened to me through the genetics I inherited from my parents?* but also *Can I understand what happened to me through the passing down genetically of the modifications my parents' genes underwent in their life experiences?* And, further, *To what extent can my own life experience then modify the way my genes are activated?*

One thorny area in epigenetics lies in the second question, of whether those alterations to your parents' gene activity can be inherited. We might inherit our parents' genes, or DNA sequences, but can we also inherit the position of our parents' genetic switches? I might have inherited a gene that is present in people with anxiety, and which was 'switched on' in my mother because of childhood trauma, but will I necessarily inherit the gene in its 'switched on' state?

Studies that have purported to show physiological effects on the grandsons of grandfathers who had experienced famine (they were less likely to have heart disease or diabetes), and on the sons of fathers who were early smokers (they had an increased risk of being above-average weight) bolster the argument that we can inherit these epigenetic features: that not only the genes themselves but the environmental effects on the expression of our forebears' genes can transmit through the generations.

But the question of epigenetic inheritance remains fraught. While multiple studies have delivered fascinating results in plants and annelids (tomatoes that pass along chemical tags that control the ripening gene; worms that pass along 'memory', in the form of a protein, that causes them to glow under ultraviolet light), we have yet to understand the mechanism supposedly behind these results in mammals. For one, it is complicated by the fact that a mammal's germ cells, the cells that become sperm and eggs, undergo a few rounds of 'reprogramming' in embryonic form, likely scrubbing away existing epigenetic markers. Epigenetic studies also focus on measuring biological markers (things like hormones, glucose) that have so many environmental influences, meaning it is very tricky to work out whether a subject's results come about through epigenetics or through in-utero exposure.

A major area of disagreement among researchers is how long the window of epigenetic change stays open. Behavioural epigeneticists claim that early life experiences can cause life-long changes to DNA. Behavioural scientist Frances Champagne at Columbia University showed that female rats licked and groomed frequently by their mothers as babies evaded male rats trying to mate with them, while those raised by inattentive mothers who did not lick and groom them allowed males to mount them.[116] Her resulting hypothesis was that the rats that are groomed have more sensitive oestrogen receptors, as a result of an epigenetic change near the oestrogen receptor gene that comes about during this early grooming. But molecular biologists and biochemists, who have been studying the mechanism behind the switching on or off of genes (a process called DNA methylation, in which chemical tags attach to the DNA to stop a gene expressing itself), have long understood DNA methylation to be something that occurs in utero and is largely fixed, and they say that studies like Champagne's are weak, over-interpreted and gloss over complex biomechanisms.[117]

If we take the idea of inherited trauma seriously, there is a third question: how do we separate out what I may have inherited from what has impacted on me in my own lived life? Can we differentiate my experiences that have caused me to be who I am from my genetic inheritance?

A similar question has been posed by the journalist Josie Glausiusz, the daughter of a Holocaust survivor and participant in what became a widely cited study of inherited trauma led by Rachel Yehuda, neuroscientist and director of the traumatic stress studies division at the Mount Sinai School of Medicine in New York.[118] Yehuda had embarked on a study investigating whether the risk of mental illness owing to trauma can be inherited, and if so whether it was passed on epigenetically, through the chemical tags that alter the way genes are expressed, rather than simply genetically, through the sequence of genes in a genome. That study had concluded that epigenetic markers in a particular area of the gene associated with the regulation of stress hormones in Holocaust survivors are capable of being passed on to the children of those survivors. In other words, the impact of trauma is heritable. But Glausiusz, who had over her childhood listened to her father, Gershon, talk about the horrors of his time in Bergen-Belsen, found herself asking, 'How does one separate the impact of horrific stories heard in childhood from the influence of epigenetics?'[119]

These inescapable problems of separating out causes are at the heart of the questions that remain in the scientific literature about whether genes play a part in perinatal depression at all. One major review of genetic influence on postnatal depression (there called postpartum depression (PPD)) concluded that, while it is known that genetics play an important role in the genesis of the disorder, the results are conflicting and in some cases need further development, especially in relation to identifying which genes are involved in PPD, and what the nature of the relationship between these genes and PPD is.[120] The authors noted: 'it seems, as in other psychiatric disorders, that genetic influence appears not to be sufficient by itself to cause the disorder. The development of psychiatric disorders is often dependent on epigenetics, and an environmental trigger is often required for these diseases to develop.'

The broader complexities of genetic studies aside, for postnatal depression research there is the extra problem of defining where the experience begins and ends. This difficulty has itself played out in the ways psychiatry has defined postnatal depression: the *DSM* has always classified it within the definition of a major depressive disorder, only acknowledging the significance of its attachment to motherhood in 1994 when the words 'postpartum onset' were added. The most recent *DSM* then expanded the parameters of the experience by changing the classification to *perinatal* depression and including pregnancy – 'during pregnancy or in the four weeks following delivery' – but postpartum support groups argue that postnatally the definition should extend to 'within six months following delivery'.[121]

The *ICD-10*, on the other hand, addresses 'mental and behavioural disorders' associated with becoming a mother according to a very specific timeframe associated with the maternal body's return to normal: the *puerperium*, or six weeks post-birth. If the symptoms of a mental or behavioural disorder emerge in these six weeks, and *if they cannot be classified elsewhere* in the *ICD*, they fall under 'code F53: Mental and behavioural disorders associated with the puerperium, not elsewhere classified'. That the *ICD-10* addresses mental experience tied to motherhood only in relation to the reproductive body and only by omission of other possible classifications reveals a curious paradox: we view the mind as somehow disembodied, and maternity as only bodied.

No doubt good epidemiological evidence to support an extended definitional timeframe will begin to emerge, and perhaps both the *DSM* and the *ICD* will change again. One Australian study, for example, concluded that 20.4 per cent of women assessed during late pregnancy and reviewed at two, four and six to eight months after the birth had an anxiety disorder (approximately two-thirds of the women with anxiety had depression, too).[122]

The question of where we begin and end a consideration of a woman's emotional experience in relation to motherhood might seem moot, but it affects treatment options: a psychiatrist considering medication for a patient with postnatal symptoms will be guided by treatment and medication recommendations that relate to the biological and practical demands of motherhood. When I eventually conceded to medication, these parameters were in a sense the crux of my predicament: was my postnatal experience part of my life story? Was it better treated with a finite course of medication or with continued psychoanalysis, or both?

For genetic research, the parameter question impacts on whether we take into account broader genetic studies on depression and anxiety to trace the heredity of PPD, or whether we consider PPD as a separate condition with its own genetic traces. Was my Paris panic, among others, connected to my postnatal experience? If it was, could I trace that more generalised depression or anxiety in me to George, and others I might not know about down the family line? If it wasn't, was it traceable to a specifically postnatal genetic trail? Fay? My own mother?

The major review I referred to earlier, on whether PPD is genetically the same as generalised depression, such as George might have had, concluded that there's not sufficient published data to determine this yet. Since that review, though, in 2016, one study investigating the relative importance of genetic and environmental influences on perinatal depression, and the genetic overlap between perinatal depression and non-perinatal depression, has come to some strong findings.[123]

In that study, two sources were investigated: the lifetime version of the Edinburgh Postnatal Depression Scale (the same test I had filled out during my Sleep School stay back when Reuben was four months old) from 3427 sets of Swedish female twins; and the clinical diagnoses of depression (separated into perinatal and non-perinatal versions) in 580,006 Swedish sisters. It is a robust study: the number of participants was high for both sources, and twin studies are considered the best source of the evidence of heritability, because they draw on the assumption that the only reason that identical twins are more similar to each other than non-identical twins is because they are more similar genetically. Through that assumption, comparisons can be made between the two kinds of twins, and genetics can be ruled in or out.

According to the study, among the twin population, genes played 54 per cent of the role in causing the subjects' perinatal depression. Environment played 46 per cent of the role. For the non-twin siblings, who would have similar but not identical genetic make-up (as the twins would) there is the expected decrease in the role genes played in perinatal depression, at 44 per cent, but this was still higher than the percentage of the role genes played in those same siblings for non-perinatal depression, at 32 per cent.

The study also showed that perinatal depression seems to constitute a subset of depression (two-thirds of the genetic contribution was shared with non-perinatal depression). Significantly, the study concluded that both kinds of depression show enough of a percentage of heritability to make them relevant to the risk and prognosis for a mother-to-be with a family history.

If we put aside the *DSM* categorising of my postnatal experience as part of a generalised depression and take it to be an acute episode of a general anxiety disorder, the data also supports a relevant percentage of heritability to my experience: twin studies of anxiety show that genetic factors contribute between 30 and 50 per cent of a person's tendency to be generally anxious or have an anxiety disorder.[124]

There was no definitive biological marker in me that was the answer to all this. My desire for such a thing was only a desire to be able to contain my experience, to gain some control over it. Freud himself, even before the explosion of our knowledge about genetics, embraced the convergence of nature and nurture in mental experience. Psychopathology 'sometimes arises more from real experiences, sometimes more from constitutional factors' he wrote, in *Mourning and Melancholia*.[125] I was not a mere robot made of bit parts and screws; my sentient mind – the part of me cultivated with my own memories and hopes and fears – could not be disregarded in this detective story.

There was another bodily aspect to be considered in my experience. How had motherhood changed me, physiologically? The obstetrician had tried to tell me about my hormonal changes just before Noah was born, but I had waded too far into my distress already to understand what was happening to me in terms of real matter; I was out on the shores of fantasy, where babies slip under rising tides and mothers are washed away.

According to emerging research on human maternal brain plasticity, new mothers undergo dynamic neural changes as they adapt psychologically to parenting and develop a bond with their infant.[126] Their brains actually change, and some of these changes place them at risk for mood disorders.

The literature on this is still limited, and the researchers behind it caution that the current data needs to be interpreted carefully until it is further replicated, but so far it shows that during pregnancy the maternal brain exhibits heightened neural reactivity in response to threats, which is considered an adaptive mechanism to protect their infant from potential danger. The problem with this is that 'hypervigilance to threats among pregnant women may also increase their vulnerability to excessive levels of anxiety and, in turn, perinatal mood disorder diagnosis'.[127]

During post-pregnancy, again as an adaptive mechanism to

strengthen the mother–infant bond, there are significant increases in activity in regions of the brain that are involved in emotion regulation, empathy and what is called maternal motivation, or desire to act in a certain way toward their child because of the pleasure associated with that behaviour. Any abnormality during this critical period of brain plasticity may increase a new mother's vulnerability to making a difficult transition to parenting: 'New mothers are exposed to a heightened level of risk for mood disorders, such as postpartum depression and anxiety disorders.'[128]

Factors such as 'mood disorders, severe stress and trauma' might disrupt what would be normal maternal brain changes, the research suggests, putting a new mother in this vulnerable position.

On the plus side, the research says that, given the high plasticity of the human maternal brain, the pregnancy and postpartum period may be one in which the maternal brain will also be highly responsive to positive interventions, such as cognitive behavioural therapy.

What of the hormonal changes the obstetrician spoke of? That our hormones go wild both when we are pregnant and postnatally is an across-the-board experience for women, necessary for the physiological changes that take place to procreate and give birth in the first place. Hormones flood the maternal body to facilitate both bonding with their baby and the necessary stress reactions to keep their baby safe. Studies on infant rhesus monkeys taken away from their mothers have shown that a mother monkey will become aggressive and show rage if their infant is removed, and in both mother and infant cortisol levels will increase.[129] Cortisol is a steroid hormone that plays a role in the body's response to stress by releasing glucose stores.

But while there have been no major differences found between the hormonal profiles of women who do and don't develop postnatal depression,[130] there remains the question of whether some may have an abnormal sensitivity to those normal physiological changes of childbirth.[131] One review looked at whether fluctuations in reproductive hormone levels during pregnancy and the postpartum period might trigger postnatal depression in susceptible women, and concluded that a certain kind of individual, with specific genetic and environmental influences, is more sensitive to postnatal hormonal changes.

The review pointed out that a major challenge to this area of research lies in formulating a study that untangles other causes of postnatal depression so that it can focus on a population in which hormonal sensitivity alone may be the cause. Many studies have therefore focused on women with postnatal depression but no prior history of major depression. The review also says that, even within this hormone-sensitive phenotype, other biological changes that take place postnatally – particularly in the immune system, the endocrinal systems, and the hormones that cause lactation – likely contribute to the development of postnatal depression.[132]

Later that week, after telling me about George, my mother stopped by with some suitcases she was lending us for the trip, and to drop off a loaf of bread, which she brought on almost every occasion she came to the house and which I had long ago determined must symbolise something, perhaps her sense of wanting me to take more of her love in, since it could not possibly be because she thought we needed bread. Gideon's hobby was baking, after all. Our bread bin was always full.

'I've got to show you something,' she said with a thrill. 'You won't believe it.' She set to work punching something into her phone, and then handed it to me. 'Lorrie sent it to me – it's a video of us from 1959. I had no idea it existed!'

A colour movie flooded the screen, people populating the camera frame in the stilted manner of mid-twentieth-century videography, looming close and then scuttling back into awkward formations as though posing for a still photograph (you could imagine instructions being shouted: *Move! Smile!*)

A little girl's face came into view and I had the uncanny feeling that I was watching Reuben: the eyes again. 'That's me!' Maxine clapped her hands gleefully. The little girl bounced up and down on her heels; it was strange to see Maxine unloosed in this child-body. And then a glamorous-looking woman, very much Jackie O, with a cigarette in her hand, a cornflower-blue cardigan buttoned over a pencil skirt, moved in behind Maxine, put her arms around her: Fay. The screen cut to black.

I felt myself well up. There was something impossible about this experience, a passing back in time to witness the locus of the thing that had been at the core of Maxine; this tenuous connection of mother and daughter that flickered in a moment on a screen. Later that night I rewound and rewound and rewound the video, which Maxine had emailed to me, trying to catch something pass between them.

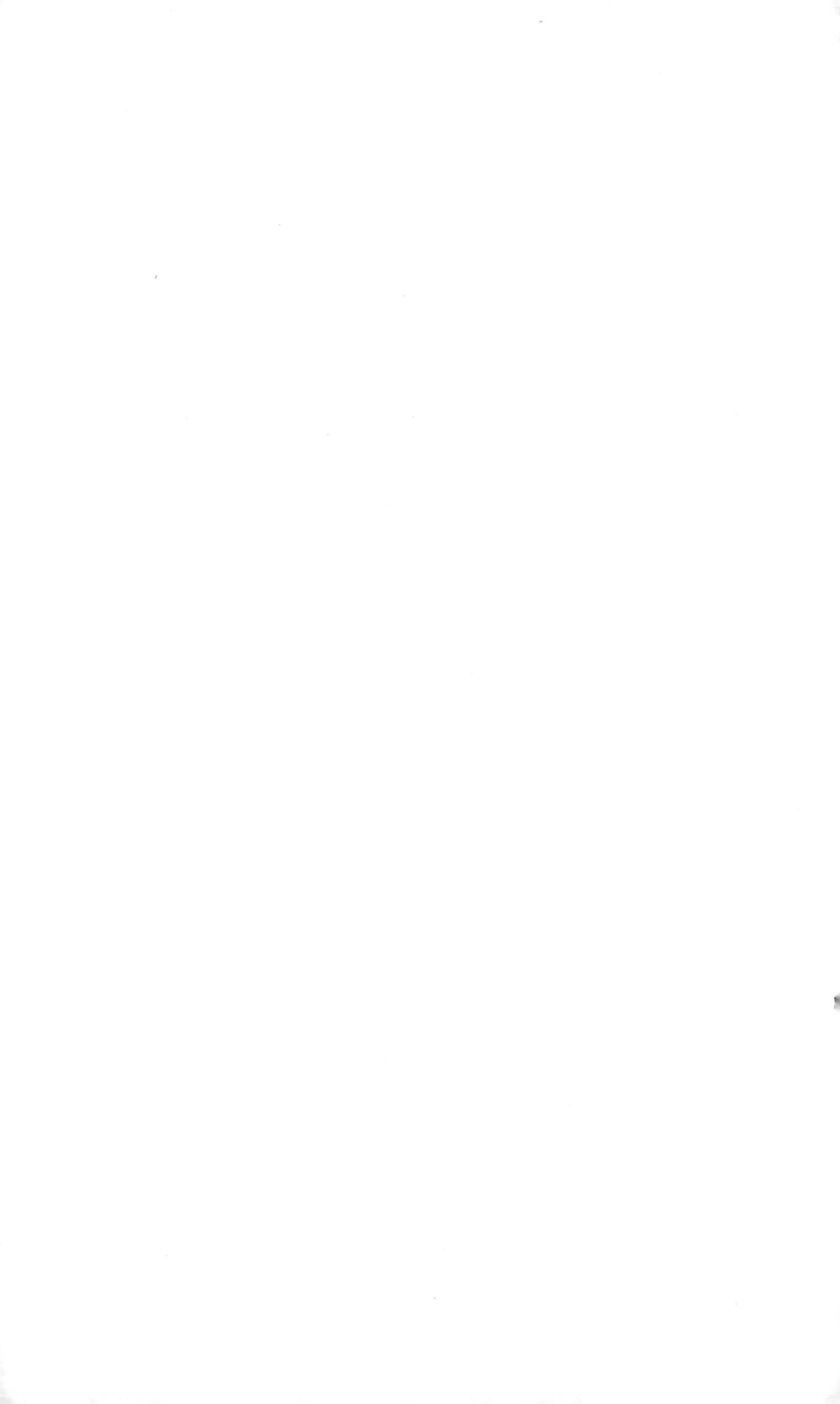

PART 3

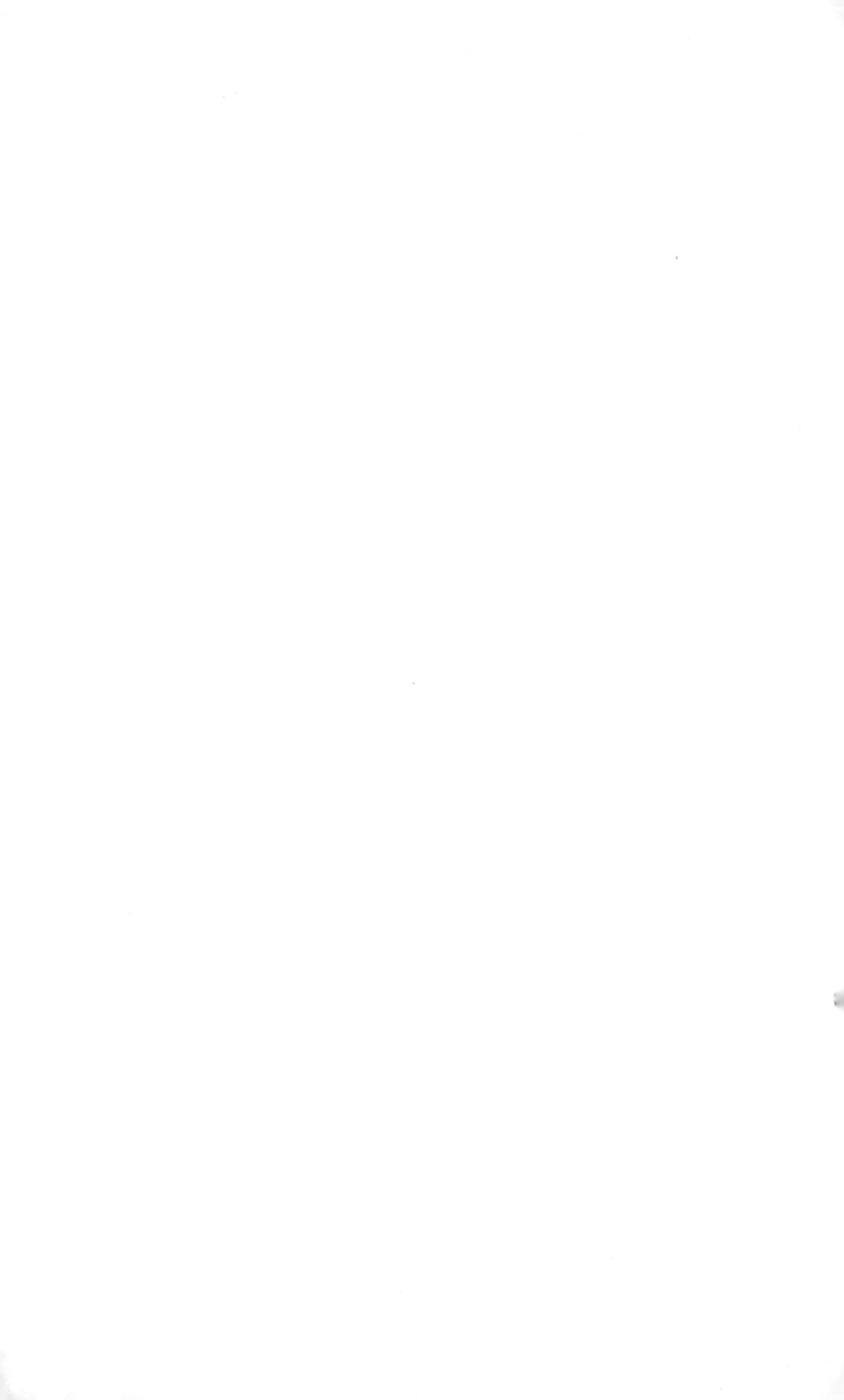

21

In the cab to the airport it was impossible for me not to think about being seventeen in my mother's car on the way to catch my flight to France. That moment, of being on the precipice of adulthood, of being unable to leap, had been the shape of me for so long. It was what I then spent the next two decades trying to undo. With Dr Parkes I had worked to find a home in myself so that I could go anywhere, go to the other side of the world, be without all my loves, and feel safe.

In motherhood, I made a home of myself twice and then had to give my babies out to the world; how hard it had been to let them leave me. Perhaps that is why the second time, with Noah, I arranged to have him cut out. My body had held on to Reuben – no amount of Syntocinon, no cervical stretching, no hook to my waters brought him out. I could not let him go.

Somewhere nearing Dubai the cabin lights flickered and Noah unfurled his limbs across me. Reuben was asleep with his head on Aaron's lap, legs on Gideon's legs. We hurtled into the darkness. I went to think of the depths of ocean beneath us, the careful physics of flight, but pulled myself back. Gideon claimed death did not scare him: 'It would be just like before you were born. Once you didn't exist, and again you won't.' But his equation only encompassed his own vanishing; it overlooked being left behind to bear the loss. I was always fighting against that liminal space of Bion's nameless dread.

Ψ

Amsterdam was glorious. It was summer; the smell of elderflowers lingered in the air, fat bees drugged themselves on the lavender blooming everywhere. We stayed in a house on a lake, near farms, out beyond the famous canals and thin buildings of the city.

There were a few days until the conference started. Gideon rode the bike paths in the sun with the children hanging off him; we ate hunks of the huge variety of breads from the supermarkets with slices of cured meat, cheeses that came in whole wheels. We let the children put the famous Dutch chocolate sprinkles on everything, because we were in Holland and nothing mattered, not even teeth.

We all slept better than we had at home, so tired from the journey and the heat and taking in the newness of things. In the mornings I found the children snuggled with Aaron playing games and being read to.

The lake glittered outside our bedroom window until late in the night when the sun finally set.

This was the Europe of my dreams.

The afternoon before the conference, Noah was restless so I put him in the pram to take him for a walk.

'Wait, I'll come with you,' Aaron called out as I was closing the door behind us.

We walked down along a path that led to the lake, where geese were dipping in and out of the water. Nothing was like Australia in summer, with its parched hardness: hyacinths and bulbs of allium exploded in gentle purples. Even the nightshades, which the owner of the house we were renting had warned us were poisonous, beckoned with softness.

'It's strange being overseas with you,' I said to him. 'The last time we travelled together I was five.' Aaron had taken Joni and me to see his family in London. Maxine still described those weeks we were away from her as the worst time of her life. Our absence had left her rudderless.

'It's wonderful,' Aaron replied. 'It makes me sad, too. It reminds me how much time we've missed together.' We walked on, bumping along a pebbled track, which began to lull Noah to sleep.

What did I know about Aaron? He was of the Beatles' generation, had grown up with the typical lifestyle aspirations of middle-class Westerners: cars and radios and pop music. He had looked like Paul McCartney and could *twist again* like a pro. He had spent his boyhood playing cricket and messing with cap guns, reading about industrious first-world adventuring with books like the *Famous Five* series. Later, at university, he was steeped in the intellectualism and artistic freedom of the 1970s, absorbing himself in theatre, the avant-garde of Beckett, revisiting modernism through TS Eliot. He had lived industrial modernity and could therefore appreciate the acuity of writers like DH Lawrence, who reflected on it. He went as far as a PhD in his education.

Going on his family background, he was far from an obvious contender for becoming a therapist, let alone a therapist of the intellectual strand of psychoanalysis. Perry, his father, whom I called by the Yiddish term *zaida*, could barely read. Perry had grown up for the first ten years of his life with only his mother – his father had taken a ship to South Africa to earn a living for the family running a concession shop on a mine. Perry followed his father to South Africa by boat from Lithuania, via England, in 1910 at the age of eleven, one of the more than two million Jews who left their villages – in what was known as the Pale of Settlement, the part of the Russian Empire to which Jews were confined – under duress of extreme persecution and discrimination.

His upbringing, education and early environment couldn't have been further from Aaron's. He had been, along with his parents and siblings, of the rural peasant class, schooled only to the age of ten. The village of his youth, Luokė, made its living from potato harvesting. He had been scurvy-riddled on that boat trip, gone quiet probably from culture shock. He, too, had run concession stores at mine sites for work, at some points of Aaron's life spending four days of the week away from home, sleeping at the store, which was far from where they lived.

When I think of Perry I think of old-world items: shoehorns and the aged leather travel pouch my father has passed on to me, which possibly once held my zaida's essential travel documents for those perilous boat journeys.

And my grandmother, Bella, her full figure and elegant jewellery outward manifestations of her status as an accomplished, competent Jewish mother – a *balabosta*, as the Yiddish term goes. Bella was technically closer in worlds to Aaron, having been born in South Africa and not in Perry's old Lithuania, from where her parents had also shipped out in the 1800s. Still, though she had changed her birth name from its original Yiddish, *Michla*, she carried with her the closed, staid silence of those old-world villages, of societies still superstitious, still locked-down in their capacity to acknowledge and speak of feelings. She had been born in the comparatively modern world of advantaged, educated white South Africa, but perhaps the real, mass tragedy that had befallen her ancestors, in pogroms and persecution, lingered in her. Perhaps feeling was innately dangerous to her. She was certainly not without her own personal tragedy: her mother had died when she was seventeen, from pneumonia. In archaic Jewish tradition her father had gone on to marry her aunt, her mother's sister, who had drowned. And then in a peculiar echo of her aunt's terrible death, her father too had died of a heart attack while swimming on a beach. (There lay another thread to be traced, this time paternally: water and its proximity to death.)

And yet. Here is the letter Bella wrote to her sister and brother-in-law on 13 January 1954 to tell them the circumstances of her father's death. It was written on a letterhead from the Hotel Empress in the seaside town of Durban, South Africa, where she was holidaying:

Dear Shira and Ilan,

Many thanks for your letter received yesterday.

We contacted the lifesaver yesterday. He came to the Empress and had drinks and dinner with us. He didn't have very much to say. He told us that Dad spoke to him about the temperature of the water, and joked over it. Then he went away, and after about a minute or two someone called him to tell him Dad was ill. He rushed straight to him and felt his pulse which was terribly slow. They quickly put him on a stretcher, and propped him as necessary, but when he felt his pulse again it had already stopped. He says they didn't wait for the ambulance then, but carried him to the Addington hospital which is over the road. He ran on first to make arrangements and as soon as the others brought Dad, the doctor immediately injected him in the heart, but nothing helped. He reckons that he had no pain and died immediately. He also said that he seemed very well liked at the *Villa Nova* and that they were all so upset that we should go see them which we shall most probably do. The lifesaver did say that immediately he died he turned blue.

Sunday and Monday it rained here and was so cold. But today it is very hot again.

With love from me and mine, Bella.

Bella never failed to describe the weather. Even in the face of her own father's death, this oddly forensic account, the corporeal detail of his turning blue, the facts of meteorology anchor the tragic news. Years later, when Aaron broke the major news to her that we were emigrating to Australia, leaving her behind, she responded with: 'Good god, Aaron; have you been eating garlic?'

You could say there was a streak of denial running through that side of the family like an arterial vein.

Ψ

With Noah fast asleep in the pram, we sat on a bench in the sun.

'You know, I think Granny Bella suffered from separation anxiety,' Aaron now told me. 'She had serious bouts of depression as an adult, and I remember one was after we moved cities for Zaida Perry's work. I was about ten. She was bedridden for six weeks. I remember being told she had hurt her back, but I knew she was depressed,' Aaron said. 'One episode we tried to convince her to see a psychiatrist, and she did, from memory, and was medicated.'

It pained me so much to slip this piece of the puzzle into my knowledge of Bella's life. I thought back to how, as a child and teenager, I would phone her from Australia, and she would always cry on hearing my voice. The distance between us all must have been unbearable for her.

'It might have started when she was a child. When she was six she was sent to a school in Pretoria, because there were no schools in the town they lived in, and she stayed with an aunt whom she hated. I think it was a terrible time for her. And then later, remember, she lost her mother at seventeen.'

So the terror of separation might have been on both sides of my family.

I felt the pull of jetlag draw my eyes closed. In that space I thought of my dream from the night before: that Aaron was at a conference in China and I had received a phone call to say he had died. 'Your father has had a heart attack in his hotel room,' the person on the other end of the phone had told me. Then I was on a train, screaming, hyperventilating with grief. *My father, my father. But I haven't told him how much I love him. But he can't be gone.* And then I was in a dark room, and in front of me were my father's belongings: a leather bag he had been carrying with him on his work trip to China. And I knew the bag contained private things that I could not bring myself to look at. Things that were to do with my father and his secrets. They took the form of slightly medical, possibly sexual objects: things to do with the body and with pleasure. Why, oh why did he die like that and leave me to deal with his bag of secrets? But, oh – the grief! I hadn't told him how much I love him!

'I just remembered I had the most awful dream about you last night,' I told him now. 'I dreamed that you died. Of a heart attack. Like Zaida Perry.'

'Oh, darling—' he reached for my hand and squeezed it.

I sniffed, trying to control the wobble I could feel rising in my voice. 'It felt so real.'

Aaron was quiet. He had a look on his face that I'd known since I was a child – his therapist look. A kind of blankness but receptiveness to his eyes. Maxine used to get angry with him when he got this look. 'Stop being a therapist and be a father,' she yelled at him one day when he dropped us back home after our weekend with him.

I knew the look well from the times when, as a child, I had asked him to show me how he used dreams in his work. On the banks of the river, surrounded by people hurling bread to the swans, he had listened with that look as I lay studiously on a blanket reaching into myself for my previous night's mind theatre.

But I wanted to do the listening today.

'I've never asked you this, but why did you became a therapist?'

In the 1950s, a book came out called *The Hidden Persuaders* by a journalist named Vance Packard. Packard, the son of a dairy farmer and his farmhand wife, became a social critic and scholar – perhaps ending as far from his origins as my father, son of a Lithuanian peasant father and homemaker, would in becoming a psychoanalytic therapist. Packard's book exposed the secret techniques of the advertising industry with a distinctly psychoanalytic subtext – 'Back to the breast and beyond' and 'Cures for our hidden aversions' were chapter titles – and somewhere in his idea of messages obscured in cigarette posters and oatmeal commercials lay the thrill of the thing that Aaron would soon find in Freud.

But then, at thirteen, Aaron had little awareness of that more academic field of human inquiry, and was mostly drawn to the way the Packard book, with its discussions of product design and shopfronts, brought a depth to something a little bit frivolous that he quite enjoyed – interior decorating. 'I was always redecorating my bedroom. I thought I'd be a window dresser. But sea matting – that was my undoing,' he told me. 'We'd been on a family holiday to Swaziland and I'd brought some home and decorated my room carefully with it. It turned out I was allergic to it. I couldn't stop sneezing.' We both became mildly hysterical at this memory of foiled refurbishment.

And then, at fifteen, another influence emboldened the effect of the Packard book on him: Manfred, Aaron's much-older sister's fiancé, who was a social worker. 'Manfred introduced me to Freud, and I realised I was interested in how the mind worked.'

The mind and its hidden persuasions. I couldn't resist putting the words of Aaron's two childhood interests side by side as a kind of answer for myself: that he became a therapist, the kind influenced by Freudian ideas of latent forces within, because he knew he was yet to confront his own secrets. That his choice of career is proof he knew there were things about himself he had not reconciled with. It's not blame I am after; not a desire to frame him. I want to know who he was before he became my father. I want to understand if he knew already he would leave me. Could that be the terror – of a father absent from my conception in heart, or mind – that lies at the centre of my anxiety? If I could come to know the answer to this, to find peace with it, perhaps it would lose its power over me.

I remembered something Maxine said when I had asked her about their marriage in the lead-up to my birth. 'I remember so clearly a thought that came to me as I drove to see the doctor early in my pregnancy with you. It was *This baby and I are going to have to make it on our own*. Maxine by then knew Aaron was on his way out.

I asked Aaron, now, when he first thought he might be gay. 'In my late teens,' he said, 'I told my brother.' Aaron's older brother, the one who had been my mother's maths tutor, arranged for my father to see a shrink. 'I lay on the couch; he was that kind of therapist.'

But that time in therapy did not resolve anything for Aaron, and whether he told Maxine of his uncertainty about his sexuality is disputed in our formal family history. Maxine maintains she had no idea; Aaron thinks he told her.

He certainly dropped a few stereotypes along the way like breadcrumbs; the window-dressing penchant, and another cliché of homosexuality that emerged in full force in his early courtship with Maxine: theatre. By the time he was beginning university he had credits in local productions of *The Merry Wives of Windsor*, *Twelfth Night*, *A Midsummer Night's Dream*, *Macbeth*, *Lysistrata* and, his *coup de grace*, the role of the Polish pianist in *Dear Friends*, which required both an accent and a semblance of piano playing. (We can at least say definitively from this evidence that Aaron was a good actor.)

And then there is this little tidbit that I can't help decoding. For his grand finale on stage Aaron set about producing his own play, choosing the Spanish dramatist Federico García Lorca's production *The Love of Don Perlimplín and Belisa in the Garden*. I looked up *Don Perlimplín*. It's a story of marital subterfuge, in which the elderly Perlimplín is convinced to marry an unsuitable younger woman, who cannot control her lust for younger men and for whom the marriage is a financial convenience. Through letters, Perlimplín woos his uninterested wife by pretending to be a younger man after her affections, and then orchestrates a duel between himself and his made-up foe. When she discovers he is the author of the letters, and that the foe does not exist, she realises she is in fact in love with her own elderly husband; that she now can feel not only lust but love – but it is too late: Perlimplín has inflicted an injury on himself as part of the act, and he dies.

It is a story rife with ambivalence about marriage – Perlimplín himself does not want to marry anyone at the start of the play ('When I was a child, a woman strangled her husband. He was a shoemaker. I can't forget it. I have always intended not to get married,' he says); Belisa, his young bride, is only satisfied by sex, not love. But by the end, Perlimplín has shed his fear of marriage and Belisa has discovered her capacity for a love based in soul not flesh.

It is also a story about hiding truths. On the marriage night, when Perlimplín is hoping to consummate his love for Belisa, two sprites enter the stage and pull grey curtains across, obscuring the audience's view. The sprites whisper to each other: 'It's always nice to cover the faults of others.'/'The audience can uncover them later.'/'Because if things are not covered with all kinds of precautions . . .'/ 'They can never be discovered.'

'Sometimes we discover too late where our passions lie,' one theatre guide gave as the précis for *Perlimplín*. In my father's production, he had Maxine operating the lighting and curtains, controlling what was revealed and concealed.

Another thing Aaron told me about his work: psychology at his university had been strongly behavioural, but he had maintained his interest in psychoanalysis and had joined the Johannesburg Psychoanalytic Society within months of its formation. There, he was exposed to the work of James and Joyce Robertson. The Robertsons had both worked for Anna Freud, Freud's daughter, when she had set up nurseries for bombed-out mothers and children in London during the Blitz. They had gone on in the 1960s to join forces with the British analyst John Bowlby to study the effects of separation on small children. The conclusions of those studies, along with their now famous recordings of the mental deterioration of a young boy named 'John' in a nursery during a nine-day separation from his mother, led to residential nurseries being closed in favour of foster care. John, who was unable to form a reliable attachment with one caregiver at the nursery and therefore failed to have his needs met adequately, grew increasingly filled with hopeless apathy as the days progressed, and showed significant aggression toward his mother when reunited with her.

At this point, Aaron and Maxine had had enough faith in their marriage to be planning their future exodus from South Africa together. Maxine was pregnant with Joni, and they agreed they would need to emigrate. Aaron had his heart set on London, but he knew he wouldn't be able to survive there on a probationary psychologist's salary while also paying the cost of analysis, which he would need to persevere with if he were to train as an analyst. They decided on Canada, where he would need a PhD to qualify to practise as a clinical psychologist.

He had been so taken by the Robertsons' studies on the effect on young children of separation from key caregivers that he decided to do his PhD in this area, studying childcare workers and the emotional impact they have on children in their care. His conclusion: high levels of empathy, authenticity and unconditional warmth have a positive influence on children's mental health.

It is a long bow to draw, but my modus operandi is to consider all connections to find meaning: was there some assurance he needed from his research about his own children's emotional needs? He was midway through the PhD when he left the marriage. For once, the implosion of personal matters overtook the looming external implosion of Apartheid, and my parents put aside talk of Canada. By the time they could think about those kinds of things again that door had closed.

Noah woke, thirsty and pink-cheeked from the afternoon sun, and we walked back along the path to the house, where Gideon was turning strings of sausages on the barbecue for dinner.

22

Aaron and I got lost trying to find the congress. It was in a university building that seemed to sprout mezzanines and sub-levels, each with unique access points from different sets of lifts. By the time we found the registration table, we were out of breath, amid throngs of similarly bewildered attendees. 'It's like being in a brain, this place, isn't it?' said a man in wire-rimmed glasses with an American accent.

We filed in to the auditorium and found our seats. 'Let's play "analyst or scientist",' I suggested to Aaron.

'Analyst,' said Aaron, as a woman with her grey hair pulled back in a low bun and clutching a string bag overflowing with papers squeezed past in the row in front of us.

Down near the lectern I spotted Mark Solms, with his wild hair and shirtsleeves. There was an air of celebrity about him, or perhaps it was only the energy of preparation: people were buzzing around him with clipboards, pinning mini microphones to themselves, sound checking.

I reviewed the program. The theme for the congress was 'Plasticity and repetition'. This referenced the neuroscientific focus *du jour* of brain plasticity, in which repeated activity has been shown to 're-wire' the synaptic connections of the brain, and the concept of repetition-compulsion – Freud's hypothesis that we strive biologically to return to earlier states of being (his 'death drive'; that we look to return to an inanimate state), which is taken by many contemporary analysts to refer to our unconscious return to attachments and behaviours set up in early life.

The speakers were a mix of psychoanalysts, some in private practice, others in research; molecular neuroscientists; affective neuroscientists; psychiatrists. Their paper abstracts spoke in the languages of psychoanalytic theory and neuroscience simultaneously, as though the two fields were not separated by the vast differences of methodological inquiry that had let Joni so easily categorise psychoanalysis as unscientific. As though neuroscience, with its objective measurables of brain regions in relation to external behaviours, might be able to sit alongside a field that asks the subjective question of what it feels like to be that brain. I was excited.

Who were these people, interested in both psychoanalysis and neuroscience? What did they want from meeting with one another? Were they here, like me, with a desire to find a point of understanding about the self that could reconcile the immaterial qualities of loss and gain and love and hate with the material of anatomy, circuitry, neurotransmitters and chemicals?

In the foyer during a tea break after two psychoanalysis-heavy papers, I spoke to a neuroscientist named Dr Samantha Brooks whose area was the neuroscience of impulse control. She studied people with anorexia and addictions. She showed me an image of the brain with various areas lit up in greens and reds, which she used on her business card: 'That's the DLPFC, the dorsolateral prefrontal cortex,' she explained. 'It helps put a stop to impulsive behaviours that come from the more primitive urges in us. And my research has found that it's turbocharged in people with anorexia,' she told me.

I wondered how her work might gel with those at the conference who would view anorexia through traditional psychoanalytic thinking, as a flight from adult sexuality with regression to phantasies and defence mechanisms. But it was time for the next panel. I took her card.

Back in the auditorium the Israeli neurobiologist Yoram Yovell had taken the stage to talk about classical neuroscientific perspectives on memory. Yovell trained with Eric Kandel, who won the Nobel Prize in 2000 for his research on the physiology of memory storage in neurons, and who had written what I found to be the most convincing argument to date about bringing psychoanalysis out from the dark of the philosophy of the mind and into the realm of science in his 1999 *American Journal of Psychiatry* article 'Biology and the future of psychoanalysis'.

Kandel had been studying history when he met and fell in love with a woman whose parents were psychoanalysts. He found a new truth in Freud's idea of the mind, but when he later took up neurobiology he found something more tenable in the clarity of scientific parameters. In his work as a neuroscientist Kandel continued to reference the Freudian construct of the mind, though he had conceded publicly that biology was a better route to the truth of man.[133]

As a Kandel protégé and trained psychoanalyst, Yovell seemed at ease using Freudian terminology like 'repression' in his overview of the neuroscience of unconscious mental processes. In his description of the famous 1911 pin-prick experiment by Édouard Claparède, which had showed an unconscious memory system at work in the amnesiac patient, he commented that the patient's withdrawal of her hand was reminiscent of Freud's transference concept: 'She knew she was afraid of him but had no idea why.' At the same time, Yovell showed no hesitation in articulating the gaps remaining in current memory research that would need to be filled to meet up with Freud's hypotheses about memory. He emphasised that, while contemporary research demonstrates that memories can become inaccessible to the conscious mind (in traumatic amnesia, for example), to align with Freud's idea of repression this kind of inaccessibility would need to be shown to be motivated – a physiological process moving toward something to fulfill a need. I listened to Yovell move between psychoanalysis and neuroscience and marvelled at how effortlessly he united the two. In this lecture theatre of accommodating minds, he could dare to proceed as though the mental and the physical could come together. What discoveries might be possible in this idyllic academic land? What insights might be won among these thinkers who had laid down their arms and come in peace?

Later, during a lengthy presentation on dream theory by a psychoanalyst, Yovell arrived late, and motioned to the empty seat beside me, which I indicated was free. Behind a lectern the psychoanalyst was putting forward an idea of dreams as a means to mental growth. He talked with as much assurance as the scientists had talked about concrete experimental findings. 'Dreams are contact barriers, like synapses,' he said. 'Dreaming is a form of thinking that focuses on seeking truth,' he went on.

Yovell was jiggling his leg up and down, I saw in my peripheral vision, and momentarily I felt his energy as disdain. But when I looked directly at him I saw something else: he was excitedly taking notes.

The story of how psychoanalysis and neuroscience came to be meeting at what was now the sixteenth neuropsychoanalytic congress begins with Mark Solms. In interviews, Solms always describes how his interest in the subjective 'I' of a person began after, as a four-year-old, he witnessed a personality change in his own brother, who suffered a traumatic brain injury at the age of six after falling from a roof. Personality changes from brain injury have long been studied in the field of neuropsychology. Probably the most famous case of such an injury was to American railroad worker Phineas Gage in 1848, when, in an explosion, a tamping iron penetrated his skull through his cheekbone and out his top cranium. Gage survived but was distinctly altered. He went from being capable and efficient to being, as his doctor noted: 'fitful, irreverent, indulging at times in the grossest profanity (which was not previously his custom), manifesting but little deference for his fellows, impatient of restraint or advice when it conflicts with his desires ... A child in his intellectual capacity and manifestations, he has the animal passions of a strong man.'[134]

What had changed in Solms's brother? The question lingered in him. Another story that comes up when Solms talks publicly about what motivated his interest in the mind: when he was six, his father told him that he no longer had to go to Sunday school, which was something Solms's mother believed in but his father did not. He could decide if he wanted to go, his father said. The choice sent the young Solms into an existential panic. What was the point of life if it ended with nothing, no heaven? Later, as an adolescent, he overcame this depression with a plan for the future: he would dedicate himself to answering the question of what it is to be a mind. 'That seemed like possibly some sort of escape out of this solipsistic nightmare,' he has said.[135]

I met with Solms the day after the congress had finished. He was juggling a full schedule as keynote speaker for his field's major annual event, and his assistant had scheduled in an early breakfast meeting for us. We located each other amid the newly laid tables of his hotel dining room.

He offered to order for me, and I watched him make his way to the counter, trying to form an early impression of the man at the centre of this academy. A wave of collegiality moved through the room with him: breakfasting neuroscientists and analysts lifted their heads from their plates and greeted him. Back at our table, he launched in to a plate of eggs and toast full bore; he had his elbows on either side of the plate, reminding me of a runner crouched low to sprint. I remembered an interview with him in which he had talked about his own experience in analysis. It had helped him see the deep guilt he had carried around with him about his brother's post-accident limitations, and in doing so freed him to fully realise his own ambitions. Perhaps it was the energy of a kind of *carpe diem* mentality I was sensing. Or perhaps it was simply confidence.

And, frankly, you'd need that in abundance to try to bring Freud into neuroscience in the twenty-first century – even to attempt to bring the study of consciousness, of feeling, into neuroscience. When Solms talked about his early motivation to do so, he was clear that his colleagues were far from encouraging; they saw it as a death knell for any future scientific career for him. 'The neuropsychology we were studying was purely cognitive – we learned about language perception, movement, all these *instruments* of the mind; but we didn't learn about the mind. And so, I started to ask my professors questions, and they were basically saying, in the nicest possible way, *You mustn't ask questions like that, that's bad for your career. We study these things; those other guys study those things.*'

Those *other guys* turned out to be the philosophy department, where students were learning about Freud, 'talking about dreams and instinctual life and phantasy, and I thought, *Wow, so here's where we can learn about that stuff*,' Solms told me. Finally, a field that treated the dynamic, mysterious source of feelings as the subject. But his timing was far from perfect, academically. It was the 1980s, and anti-Freudian sentiment was at a peak. The neuroscientist J Allan Hobson had metaphorically danced on Freud's grave with his research that claimed to show, contrary to Freud's elaborate hypothesis of dreams as meaningful mind work, that dreams are nothing more than random neural activity. Solms was undeterred. He formed a mission: to bring the 'outside' study of the brain and correlating behaviours and the 'inside' study of the mind and correlating feelings into one field. As he put it in a 2015 interview in *The Atlantic*: 'There can't be a mind for neuroscience and a mind for psychoanalysis. There's only one human mind.'[136]

Facing being drafted into the army, Solms left South Africa for the UK, where he took a position as a neuropsychologist at the Royal London Hospital, working with brain-injured patients, and at night trained as a psychoanalyst. In his work in acute care and rehab, he began to bring the two areas of practice together.

'It was where the patients actually lived – you got to know them as people; you got to see how they related to each other and to the staff. I started to sit and talk to the patients, and to try to get to know them as people,' he explained to me.

Solms recognised that there had been significant technological advancements in neuroscience since Freud's time, and that the study of the mind in relation to brain injury (clinico-anatomical correlation), which Freud had abandoned shortly after his paper on aphasia, might now be able to draw on the hypotheses of psychoanalysis to continue where Freud left off. To do so, though, would require acknowledging what Solms says neuroscience has avoided broaching: the fact that the brain is not an organ like the liver or the lungs. That it possesses the special property of consciousness, which means it possesses subjectivity.

According to Solms, we therefore have two sources of data about the mind: objective observation of the brain and behaviour, and that which science has so far shunned: 'the raw data provided by … introspective reports', or the subjective observations of a person concerning their current mental experiences.

But much occurs in our minds, or our introspective experience, that we do not perceive. (What, for example, occurs to cause a long-forgotten memory to arrive in our thoughts?) For Solms, this is why psychoanalysis offers the best scientific method for considering the mind: because it accounts for events that occur in these gaps in internal perception (or that which is unconscious). Since psychoanalysis considers such gaps to be mental as much as it considers conscious thought to be mental, says Solms, it constructs about the mind 'a universe of natural phenomena (a complete chain of cause and effects) that can be studied scientifically like any other aspect of nature'.[137]

One important proviso to Solms's outlook: the brain should be regarded as dynamic, much as Freud had envisaged. It is not a static organ with modular functions, like a car engine. Rather – and here Freud took on the work of a figure relatively under-celebrated in the popular annals of brain study, the Soviet neuropsychologist Alexander Romanovich Luria – the brain is understood as a connected set of functional systems that work in groups, and the mind resides within those dynamic systems. Luria had, for example, understood speech and language production as a sequence of neurological processes happening in connected parts of the brain, so that inner language was turned into semantic representations in one part, then into semantic structures in another, then into syntactic structures in another, and finally into speech in yet a different part. By understanding the brain as complex connected systems, Luria offered a concept of the mind's working that addressed the intricate abstract process that mental activity is, in which, as Solms describes: 'Simple mental functions have widely distributed physical correlates … mental functions can never be found *inside* neuroanatomical structures; they exist, as it were, *between* them.'[138]

The mind, in this way, according to Solms, does not have direct correlates in localised brain tissue. There is mental experience (subjectively perceived feeling); there is the organ of the mind (the brain); and, inferred from the two, there is mental apparatus (a virtual thing, a model; what exists *between* the neuroanatomical structures). My postnatal experience existed dynamically in my mind: it lingered between memory and cognition and my language apparatus and every other aspect of my self that made me sentient. There could be no pin-drop on my brain to locate a feeling or thought or experience.

If you consider that the mind 'carries within itself the whole of its developmental history', as Solms put it, and that every perception experienced, internal or external, involves dynamic references to other mental experiences (memories, for one), you can see why psychic reality can never be pinned down to material reality, and why 'it would be foolish to believe that we will ever explain the psychological reality of mental illness by means of anything other than psychology'.[139]

Was there any way, then, to better delineate the systems at work in the brain that organise what makes us sentient? Solms felt sure, after his work at the Royal London Hospital, that it might be possible to finally make the study of subjective mind states a viable area of science if we could bring the psychoanalytic method (offering its complete chain of cause and effects, as Solms felt it did) to the subject of brain injury. Along with his primary collaborator Karen Kaplan-Solms (also his wife), much of his work in the late 1990s then aimed, in his own words, to 'draw broad brushstrokes' in an attempt to make anatomical descriptions relate to basic psychoanalytic concepts.[140]

He described it in this way in a 2002 paper: 'We study patients with damage to circumscribed parts of their brains, just as cognitive neuroscientists do. We try to understand how their minds are altered by the changes in their brains. However, the method that we use to make our clinical observations and the theory that we use to organize those observations are psychoanalytical.'[141]

What Solms says he is not trying to do is reduce the mental to the physical. Rather, his point is that 'the mind is no less real than the brain', and in the case of damage to a specific part of the brain, neuropsychoanalysis offers a way to understand the material and the psychic together. It says that a model of cause and effect that explains a person's inner emotional experience (psychoanalysis), correlated with a physical site of injury, will begin to show us an architecture of the mind.

Take, for example, Solms's study of patients with right-hemisphere damage: the patients all revealed to him in different ways, through their communications, varying psychological responses to how their bodies had been affected by their brain injury. Some seemed to reject their now paralysed limbs, while others obsessed over them. Solms understood their psychological reactions in terms of Freudian ideas of defences: they either 'forgot' the affected limb or demanded its removal. These were, he concluded, defensive coping mechanisms to deal with the painful feelings of damage to their sense of their bodies in the world. Their choice of defensive mechanism differed because of their individual life histories (since in Freudian theory we repeat our emotional responses according to how we first experienced the same kind of trauma as an infant).

Patients with left-hemisphere damage who suffer limb paralysis, Solms argued, do not display these defences. They make 'realistic adaptations' to their injuries. Why would this be the case? Solms's answer contains the next step in bringing together the psychical and the material. While the right hemisphere affects the representation of 'things' in our mind, so that if damaged our spatial sense of our bodies in the world collapses, the left hemisphere affects 'symbolic representations of the body' only (the lexicon and semantics of how we represent our bodies in speech, for example). In this way, left-hemisphere patients (because while losing their words they retain a concrete sense of their body as an object) do not forget or disown their injured body parts in the way that right-hemisphere patients do, which means they are able to go through the 'necessary process of mourning' their injury.[142]

'So that kind of study has a purpose for a brain-injured patient beyond what *you* learn from it scientifically?' I asked him.

'The ethical principle upon which the whole of psychoanalysis is based is that it's always better to know the facts. Why? Because they're there,' he told me, mopping up his egg yolk with a piece of toast. 'If you don't know them and they're there, you're going to bang into them, and you're going to get a bloody nose. The more primitive our defences are, the less successful they are at actually helping you to meet your needs in the world. So as much as it might appear to be cruel to try to persuade a patient to face unpleasant realities, I think it is helpful. That doesn't mean that you can cure them, but it's helpful. The other way that it's helpful is for the family to better understand what's going on so they react more appropriately to the patient.' If Phineas Gage had been around these days, he may have lain on Solms's couch and found some consolation in having his aggressive thoughts understood as unconscious desires.

Solms's papers from this time make for fascinating reading, offering the tantalising hope that something meaningful can be made from the words and communications of the profoundly brain-injured, and that an injured brain can offer us a scientific opportunity for the study of emotion. In his 2002 study of a patient with Korsakoff's syndrome, which he described as 'a very bizarre, disturbing alteration of personality that occurs when there are lesions in front of the third ventricle', Solms uses a psychoanalytic framework to address what has gone wrong with the functional structure of the patient's mind and, conversely, to understand what that part of the mind does in a person. Korsakoff's syndrome results in a profound amnesia with what's called a temporal gradient (meaning the patient's ability to remember is weaker the newer the memory is – they can't lay down new memories, and the more recent a memory pre-onset the more vulnerable it is to being lost) along with the strange behaviour of confabulation, in which the person maintains false beliefs and invents stories to address what they cannot explain on account of the memory loss. Solms treats the patient's confabulations not as nonsense but as material that can be understood as unconscious desires and wishes: the repressed, the transformed, the symbolic.

Take this vignette as narrated by Solms, in which the patient, a former electrical engineer, who is unaware of what has happened to his mind but is distressed by his own confusion, refers to terminology he has retained from his working days: '[The patient] says, "I think the problem is a cartridge is missing. We must … we just need the specs," by which he means specifications. "We just need the specs. What was it? A C49? Should we order it?"

'I say, "What does a C49 cartridge do?"

'He says, "Memory. It's a memory cartridge, a memory implant."'

Rather than dismiss the patient's words as the spouting of random mind flotsam, Solms takes them seriously as meaningful emotional representations and uses the moment to facilitate understanding for him: 'I say to him, "You're aware that something's wrong with your memory but—" and he interrupts me and says, "Yes, it's not working 100 per cent, but we don't really need it."

'... I think it is really an enormous step forward for him to recognize that his memory isn't working, let alone knowing that we are talking about memory at all.'[143]

Recalling this case study, I asked Solms how he felt about the hurdle of getting empirically minded scientists to regard his interpretations of a patient's emotional representations as hard data. He explained his methodology in more detail: 'There is an ordinary person sitting there talking rubbish and he's got all kinds of weird ideas about C49 and his cartridge that we have to order, so that's the qualitative lived experience – the kind of thing a natural scientist would think is just nonsense, just words. But you get the feeling there's some meaning to this; why is he using that image rather than this one? And then you see certain regularities: there's no question this is distorting reality in a tendentious way to make things better, for example. Then you can start, as we did, to apply objectivity. We took the first 150 confabulations in a consecutive series and we gave them to blind raters who had to rate them on an affect scale, and that shows, *Well, yes, he makes it better*, and then we took ten such patients, and said, *Okay, was it just this patient or was it all of them?* Then you say, *Okay, now we've got a regularity; this is an objective finding.* Then you can start saying, *What is it about that lesion? What part of the brain is it damaging that is performing which function that seems to have an inhibition of wish-fulfilment role?* And it turns out to be this ventro-medial frontal cortical area, and then you can say, *What does it connect to? How does it grow in development? What is the chemistry? How does it look in other animals?* and next thing you are down to a molecular level, and there's a seamless continuity.'

By taking seriously the emotional life of the patient, and of the other Korsakoff's syndrome patients Solms studied with Kaplan-Solms, he came to conclude that '[Korsakoff's] is not simply a cognitive defect. There is an emotionally based factor too which accounts for the symptoms ... one is seeing ... not simply a deficit of the machinery of memory. There is something that *rises up* to fill the gap left by that deficit ... there is a dynamic interplay. The reality-monitoring part of the mind is weakened, and some other force, which is usually held at bay, rises up ...'[144]

This was where I thought the crux of Solms's hypothesis was to be found, and where you could witness his real defence of psychoanalytic theory through anatomical mapping. He proposed in that paper, looking cumulatively at the Korsakoff's patients he and Kaplan-Solms studied, that the 'other force' that 'rises up' in those patients' minds has four particular qualities, and those qualities match up with the four functional features of the unconscious that Freud put forward in his seminal paper 'The unconscious'.

First, they replace external reality with a psychical reality (for example, patients spoke of their previous night's dreams as actual events that took place). Second, their thinking is exempt from mutual contradiction (for example, one patient believed that the man in the bed next to hers was her husband, but she also recognised her husband when he visited her, and when both men were present she accepted them as both being her husband). Third, they lack a sense of time as an objective entity (for example, one patient always believed it was 5 pm even in the face of contradictory evidence). Fourth, they engage mainly in the more primitive state of thinking (known as primary-process thinking) that Freud believed unconscious thought came from (for example, the patient for whom the C49 cartridge was his memory).

What does a conclusion like this, about a specific group of patients with a particular localised brain lesion, mean more broadly for a theory of the mind? According to Solms, it offers 'a foothold in functional anatomy, in order to link our basic psychoanalytical concepts with the functional anatomy of the brain'. In other words, it begins to form an understanding of the architecture of the mind. Put together with studies of other syndromes arising from different kinds of brain-injuries, it would cumulatively begin to give us 'a better theory of how the mind works, which is ultimately the aim of both neuroscientists and psychoanalysts'.[145]

Neuropsychoanalysis is not only this clinico-anatomical work of discovering the causal mechanisms of emotional symptoms. It also takes up specific questions of mind–brain function, many of which were Freud's starting points: what, for example, is the function of dreams? This had been a focus for Solms, whose research into the neurological underpinning of dreaming challenged the longstanding research of neuroscientist J Allan Hobson, which had concluded dreams were meaningless images, the result of chemical activations during rapid eye movement (REM) activity. Hobson's conclusions pivoted on dreaming being confined to REM sleep,[146] but Solms's data showed dreams can occur outside REM sleep, and facilitated a model of the mind that reframed dreams as 'motivated phenomena, driven by our wishes', much as Freud had said.[147]

Was Solms hoping to prove Freud right? I wondered, thinking of Joni and how she once said to me, 'Science should proceed without bias toward a given result.' His aim, he explained to me, was never to do anything for psychoanalysis, but rather to do something for neuropsychology with psychoanalysis. 'But in the process of acquainting myself with what Freud was all about I realised that a great disservice had been done to him.' Psychoanalysis, in being the only field dedicated to what Solms calls 'a great neglect of the subjective, sort of sentient motivated agent of the mind' offered an obvious starting point for his work, and has provided rich conceptual frameworks for his discoveries, even beyond Freud.

'Psychoanalysts get irritated with me, saying, *Why is it all this Freud, Freud, Freud?* and *Psychoanalysis didn't end with Freud; why don't you use my favourite theory?* but they're missing the point of what it is that we've come to do. I've found that I've had to borrow concepts even beyond Freud: for example, in anosygnostic patients [who seem unaware of their brain-injury and confabulate reasons for their situation], people like Melanie Klein lend much better conceptual sort of explanatory terminologies and ideas in her notions of splitting and projections and those primitive sorts of defences.'

Along the way, Solms had also ended up proving Freud wrong. 'There inevitably are times when you find, *But hang on, this doesn't fit.* As we make advances in neuropsychoanalysis in better understanding how the mind works, so it will inevitably have implications for psychoanalysis too,' he told me.

If there was a revolution being staged by neuropsychoanalysis, it was in Solms and his colleagues saying that these emotionally based dynamic forces that rose up in those Korsakoff's patients, or right-hemisphere-injured patients, and that rise up in dream material or other brain outputs, need to be taken seriously as subjects of scientific study. That it is not enough to say feelings cannot be studied scientifically because they only exist subjectively. For Solms and his colleagues, feelings, as reported experiences of consciousness, cause behaviour and can be studied objectively as such, much as learning can be studied objectively in the field of behaviourism.

Here is how he put it, in a 2010 article he co-wrote with affective neuroscientist Jaak Panksepp: 'Feelings evolved for good biological reasons; they make specific, concrete contributions to brain functioning ... we must admit that consciousness actually exists, that it is a property of nature.'[148] To ignore consciousness and the subjective experience of feelings, according to Solms and Panksepp, ignores the possibility that feelings have a functional biological role.

'But how *do* you go about studying feelings, consciousness, scientifically?' I asked Solms.

He pointed over to a table not far from us, where a man whom I recognised as Panksepp from his seminar the day before, white-bearded and elfin, was chatting with other attendees. 'You've got to talk to Jaak. I mean, that's the story of his life. He wanted to study emotion, feeling, to understand what it is as a natural scientist,' Solms told me.

But I didn't get to talk to Jaak, who left his table before I had finished talking to Solms. By the time I got around to understanding the implications of his work, he had passed away unexpectedly.

My time with Solms came to an end. He had to get to the airport. He left the dining room still greeting people, laughing, and I was again struck by his palpable *joie de vivre*. Perhaps that's what came of not fearing emotion and its meaning. I remembered now that Solms ran a vineyard back in Cape Town – Solms-Delta, a family inheritance. According to the business's website, he had returned to overhaul the vineyard after Apartheid ended, but had come up against hostility from the seven households of people who had been tenants on the land for generations, building up his family's estate essentially as slaves. Solms's remedy was much like the psychoanalytic method: unearth their stories, acknowledge their reality. The vineyard now has an historical museum of artefacts in recognition of its past, and ownership is split 50/50 with the tenants.

I waited at the table for Aaron to return from exploring the canals of Amsterdam, still thinking about Solms and his work. He had his detractors: psychology researcher G William Domhoff had made a case against him for misunderstanding the history of the REM controversy 'in a Freudian-serving way' and ignoring 'the considerable systematic empirical evidence that contradicts the key claims of the Freudian dream theory he is trying to revive'.[149] 'Domhoff is from the generation that was kind of traumatised by the psychoanalysts having the truth,' Solms had said to me when I had mentioned him.

There was J Allan Hobson, too, who had penned a number of rebuttals to Solms's work, including one titled 'In bed with Mark Solms? What a nightmare!' Hobson is famous for his anti-Freudian stance that dreams do not offer concealed symbols: 'In dreams, what you see is what you get,' he wrote in a *Scientific American* article called 'Freud returns? Like a bad dream'.[150]

And there was other, surprising, opposition to Solms and neuropsychoanalysis: a faction of psychoanalysts who believed Solms and his colleagues were not in the service of strengthening the authority of the field, but undermining it. Psychoanalysis must be studied hermeneutically not scientifically, in their view. Marshall Edelson, psychiatrist and author of a book in the late 1980s arguing for scientific rigour in psychoanalysis, said that to look to biology to provide this would be conceptually impossible as the two fields share no common language or conceptual framework, and 'should be resisted as expressions of logical confusion'.[151]

A more recent case against neuropsychoanalysis was put comprehensively in an article by that title in the *International Journal of Psychoanalysis* in 2007, by Rachel B Blass and Zvi Carmeli from the psychology department at the Hebrew University of Jerusalem, which has spurred a series of responses and counter-responses. Neuropsychoanalysis, Blass and Carmeli say, reflects a pervasive trend in Western culture toward biologism: 'that what is real is biological ... [that] our thoughts and experiences as subjective psychological entities are secondary and ephemeral relative to the concrete reality of tangible neural structures'.[152] They believe it is unhelpful to psychoanalysis to turn to neuroscience, which 'ascribes to biology a kind of significance that does away with the value of meaning and psychic truth which is at the foundation of psychoanalysis'.[153] The only instance in which they see neuroscience as helpful to psychoanalysis is in its ability to identify where a person might have a neuronal injury or abnormality that would, according to Blass and Carmeli, prevent them engaging in psychological intervention.

Even if a neuroscientific finding overthrows an assumption at the heart of the psychoanalytic method, Blass and Carmeli say it is irrelevant to the experience of analysis and its potential outcomes, which rely on a specific subjective experience of meaning-making. To argue, for example, about whether apparently forgotten traumatic memories can be retrieved accurately or at all (neuroscientific findings have shown that memory is labile, both able to be manipulated and introduced) misses the fact that the analytic process turns on the imagined more than the actual lived experience. Freud, after all, had written of the 'difficulty in distinguishing unconscious phantasies from memories which have become unconscious'.[154]

Likewise, to try to prove that dreams do indeed arise biologically in the exact manner Freud proposed is, say Blass and Carmeli, quite irrelevant to whether or not meaning may be found in the dream material during the analytic process: 'to speak of neuroscience and psychoanalysis as two irreducible perspectives on human experience would be like considering chemistry and art as two irreducible perspectives on the paintings of Van Gogh. Indeed there would be no painting without the chemical components of paint and canvas, but to suggest that these components provide an explanation of the painting that would be valuable for the artists is to deny the value of art.'[155] To continue to look to neuroscience to validate psychoanalytic work, in Blass and Carmeli's view, undermines the real value of the psychoanalytic process, which is to arrive at meaning.

Yoram Yovell, Mark Solms and their colleague Aikaterini Fotopoulou penned a response to Blass and Carmeli, in which they reasserted the aim of neuropsychoanalysis as an attempt to 'build a bridge' between neuroscience and psychoanalysis rather than to merge the two or usurp one with the other.[156]

Their position is perhaps captured best by Eric Kandel, who argued in his seminal 1999 paper that neuroscience and psychoanalysis have differing aims and perspectives and only converge at points, and that biology cannot address the scope and complexity of psychoanalysis: 'The role of biology in this endeavour is to illuminate those directions that are most likely to provide deeper insights into specific paradigmatic processes.'[157] At the same time, they are firm on this: an acceptance of dual-aspect monism, that the mind and brain are one, is the only sensible way forward for either field, and that to deem it otherwise – as Blass and Carmeli seem to do – will only serve to diminish the relevance of psychoanalysis today.

There is a Latin saying about alcohol and disinhibition: *in vino veritas* (in wine, truth). A vineyard, too, is a scientific venture. But what it reaps can be understood in multiple ways depending on where you stand on the matter of such things: it is to harvest chemicals that will be imbibed; it cultivates nature; it is merely a business.

23

Jaak Panksepp, the man Mark Solms had suggested I speak to, was known as 'the rat tickler'. In the 1970s, he'd discovered that rats chirped when engaged in the rat equivalent of tickling – rough play with a human hand – and he was certain that the sound was a vocalisation of joy.

Why was he tickling rats in the first place? He had begun his career studying psychology in the hope of learning about human emotion, but found himself in the thick of behaviourism, where only observable stimulus-response experiments were counted. Emotion was considered well outside the parameters of objective observation. In an electroencephalography lab, studying brain waves as part of his PhD, he became excited by the technique of brain-stimulation reward, where electrodes are placed in the brain to generate a pleasurable feeling.

The king of behaviourism, BF Skinner, had recently established a learning process called operant conditioning, in which a subject experiences a particular stimulus directly after enacting a behaviour, and in that way develops a learned response to the stimulus. Skinner's work built on that of Edward Thorndike, who a century earlier had developed his 'law of effect': that a behaviour which elicits pleasure will be repeated, and one that elicits displeasure will be stopped. A rat, for example, who receives the reward of food after pressing a lever, will return to press the lever. A rat given an electric shock after pressing a lever will in future avoid the lever. James Olds and Peter Milner, shortly after

Skinner, took Skinner's findings deep into the brain, showing in rats the physiological basis of operant conditioning by locating a 'reward' centre in their brains that could be stimulated using electrodes. The rats continually pressed the lever that turned the electrodes on.

In his lab, Panksepp was conducting this same kind of experiment with rats, but he was thinking about what he observed in a way that was virtually taboo in his field: that the display signs of his rats were emotional. That the electrodes provoked rat joy, and that those reward and punishment centres in the rats' brains were more than on/off buttons for behaviour: they were the neurobiological sites of emotion.

A century earlier, Darwin had hypothesised that emotion had an evolutionary basis. In *The Expression of the Emotions in Man and Animals* (1872), he said that humans and some animals show emotion through similar behaviours, and that these displays evolved over time. A number of neuroscientists had taken Darwin's ideas further in the human realm, looking at the evolutionary bases of emotion, but the overarching scientific view remained that it was pointless to suppose emotion in other animals.

Panksepp was determined to forge ahead with an hypothesis of animal emotion, despite a critical reception from his peers – 'I brought up the psychological issues, and my professor said, *Panksepp, I've seen guys like you before, and they're not around anymore*,' he told *Discover* magazine in 2012 – and soon enough he hit on his next most significant finding.[158] This time, the experiment involved a lever that the rat could press to stimulate their medial forebrain bundle. The rats repeatedly pressed the lever, which was a simple enough sign that the lever elicited pleasure for them, much the way that rats in another of his experiments had demonstrated their pleasure by returning to press a lever that fed them sugar water.

But Panksepp noticed that the behavioural display of the brain-stimulated rats was not quite the same as it was when they were delivered the sugar-water reward. Those rats had displayed relaxed behaviour, and had stopped returning for sugar water when they were full. But the brain-stimulated rats displayed energetic exploration of their surroundings after a jolt, and did not stop pressing the lever. He decided to wire rats up to electrical-brain stimulation that *also* delivered a shot of sugar water to their stomachs. The rats kept showing this purposeful, seeking exploration, and they kept pressing the lever even when their stomachs were completely full. In fact, they returned to do so right up until they killed themselves from overfilling their stomachs.

What was this energised, expectant seeking that Panksepp was seeing in the brain-stimulated rats? Why was the feeling so compelling that it overrode the displeasure of their physical fullness? Panksepp concluded that the medial forebrain bundle represented a different, and highly significant emotional system; one that set off a foraging kind of behaviour in animals, an excitement, a goading. An in-built exploratory system designed to generate expectancy and *motivation to seek* in the mammal. He named this the SEEKING system. The SEEKING system gets 'thirsty animals to water, hungry animals to food, cold animals to warmth'.[159] (All of Panksepp's affect systems are spelled out in upper case to differentiate them from other uses of the same words.)

'Expectancy' and 'motivation to seek' are not behaviours. They are affects – Panksepp's term for emotions – and in this way his work went out of the bounds of behavioural science. Panksepp was of the firm belief that displays of affect could not only be clearly identified but were absolutely necessary aspects of psychological study, and of biological study. Affective feelings, in Panksepp's paradigm, which are 'within-brain' feelings, had biological purpose, much like sensory affects (sensations from outside the body, like burning heat on your hand or the smell of a flower) and homeostatic affects (sensations from inside the body, like hunger or tiredness). They were tools for living that allowed an animal to survive, and they were guided by past learning, internal bodily regulation and external, real-world incentives.

Over the next years, he turned his focus to identifying these in-built systems of affect, or emotion, in mammalian brains – systems he called *primary processes* – and on mapping their neural networks, resulting in another six additional 'core mammalian emotions': RAGE, FEAR, LUST, CARE, PANIC/GRIEF and PLAY. He proposed that these neural systems, deep in the brain, give us our basic tools for living by providing us with feelings that tell us if an act is rewarding or punishing, and trigger a set of behavioural responses to optimise survival. PLAY, for example, provides a system that allows mammals to discover the rules of their social world in a joyful way.

The PANIC/GRIEF system, on the other hand, 'evolved for the purpose of mediating attachment and loss, and ... produce[s] the particular type of pain associated with these biological phenomena of universal significance – namely, *separation distress* ... which, if it does not result in reunion, is typically followed by hopeless despair'.[160] Panksepp saw the purpose of these feelings as to motivate the mammal to seek reunion with their lost mother/group/sexual partner and, if they could not do so, to eventually give up and fall into despair. An animal wailing in distress, after all, is vulnerable to attack by predators. Despair, which brings with it lack of motivation to forage, to cry out, to seek, is a safer option for an animal unable to defend itself alone in the wild. The pain the animal feels, therefore, has *biological value*. (I could not but wonder how my PANIC/GRIEF system operated: perhaps the neural systems that caused those feelings in me worked in overdrive.)

Panksepp saw the seven systems as fundamentally interactive, so that like systems would facilitate each other and opposing systems would inhibit each other. Among the systems, SEEKING, which describes an urge to obtain a goal, and motivates organisms to act, is ever-active, working with at least one of the other six systems, so that the organism has a goal that they are motivated toward (in the PANIC/GRIEF case, for example, neural mechanisms during what he calls the despair phase shut down the SEEKING system, so that the animal does not forage or look for water and put itself in danger).

Are Panksepp's emotional systems equivalent to Freud's drives, our unconscious strivings toward pleasure and pain, life and death? Not quite. Freud's drives, after all, were unconscious. Panksepp's systems must be *felt* or they have no purpose. Unlike Freud's 'primary processes' – which was the term he used to describe unconscious mental processes that took place in the id – Panksepp's primary processes are a primitive form of consciousness. We *feel* them, and we need to feel them so they can play their necessary biological role in our survival.

What is unconscious, Panksepp argued, is the next layer up of our brain processes, which provides life experiences that modify our instinctive systems: our learning and memory-formation. 'Thinking can be repressed, but emotions cannot,' explained Brian Johnson and Daniela Flores Mosri, in their wide-ranging overview of the neuropsychoanalytic approach.[161]

And after that layer, Panksepp said, is the layer of our brain, the cortex, that is fully conscious, where we form thought and make plans, and which in humans is far bigger than it is in animals.

Part of the basis for Panksepp's belief that his primary-process systems are in-built and of biological purpose was that all the systems he mapped out were located in the deep subcortical regions of the brain. For Panksepp, who had embraced a contentious evolutionary theory of the mammalian brain, that it evolved in a series of distinct structures that emerged from the primitive 'reptilian brain' at its core, the existence of these affective systems in that initial brain structure was evidence that the systems had intrinsic biological purpose:

> Primary processes … manifest evolutionary memories that are the basic emotional operating systems of the brain. Secondary processes … are enriched with the mechanisms for learning – for linking external perceptions with associated feelings. Then on top, the tertiary level is programmed by life experiences through the neocortex, engendering our higher cognitive processes such as thinking, ruminating, and planning. Our capacity to think is fueled by our storehouses of memory and knowledge acquired by living in complex physical and social worlds.[162]

His brain map and theory of mammalian emotion was against the grain of traditional brain sciences. For one, it has been a long-held view in neurology that higher brain functions, in the neocortex and cortex, where perception and thinking happen, govern emotional experience and consciousness. The basis for behavioural neuroscience, for example, has been that behaviour gives way to learning. Panksepp disagreed: affects – internal feeling states – which originate in brain-stem and subcortical circuits low down, and which are *felt*, are for him the foundation of consciousness, and give way to higher cognitive learning. Indeed, it is well-established that consciousness is obliterated when the upper brain stem is damaged, while removal of most of the cortex has a far less expansive effect on consciousness.[163] The circuits Panksepp mapped, which aroused the particular emotional states that gave rise to the names of his seven systems, generate conscious feeling states that are internally categorised as either good or bad for us, serving to promote our chances of survival. This is what consciousness is for, he said.

Many other brain researchers have brought to light this connection between emotional feeling and cognition, dispelling the idea that we operate with a disconnect between our reasoning and our feeling. Neuroscientist Antonio Damasio demonstrated that we cannot, in fact, live our lives without the feeling states that guide us toward decision-making. Damasio famously made his case for this in his book *Descartes' Error*, in which he described a patient named Elliot who had frontal lobe damage. Elliot performed well on intelligence tests, but could not make good life decisions, manage time, assess good character. It turned out Elliot could not feel emotions either. When shown gruesome images he was aware they were designed to elicit strong emotion in him but he did not know what that emotion was. He felt neutral. His impaired affect had impaired his ability to make his way in life. It made it impossible for him to prioritise, be motivated, choose. Emotional feeling, according to Damasio, is a necessary biological event.[164]

In Panksepp's paradigm, the core mammalian instincts, deep in the subcortex, are necessary not only for emotion to be felt but for memory and thinking in our higher brain to be formed: 'ancient feeling states help forge our memories in the first place. New memories could not emerge without the underlying states that allow animals to experience the intrinsic values of life,' he once explained.[165]

I recalled now the neuroscientist Samantha Brooks, who had shown me the image of the dorsolateral prefrontal cortex, and how she had described a higher-up part of the brain, a cognisant part, that *helps put a stop to impulsive behaviours that come from the more primitive urges in us*. She had been describing what Panksepp was describing. Anorexics, she had found, had super-strong working memories in their higher brain. That part was literally stamping on their bodies' desire. (My lists, lists, lists, of food and feeding times and sleeping times.) Why might it do this? And was the brain doing this because the brain was an anorexic brain, born with that kind of functioning? Or did it develop into that sort of brain because of life experience? When I later wrote to Brooks, she told me that, beyond her clinical work, she had begun to think about an hypothesis she had read of anorexia as a disorder of the 'development of the self':

> I think … that anorexia is rather about an inability to cope with one's subjective experience, because one's self has not developed separate enough from one's primary care giver in the early stages of life ([in the vein of] psychoanalytic attachment theories of Bowbly, Winnicott etc.) … This makes intuitive sense to me. And since the separate self does not develop sufficiently in a person who goes on to have anorexia, there is an over-reliance on cognitive – as opposed to affective – responses to the environment in order to guide one's decisions … it could be that cognitive deficits are expressions of a deficit in the development of the self, expressed neurobiologically.[166]

Much of Panksepp's work, right up until his death, was only accepted among a minority in his field, and his detractors remain. For one, the idea of mammalian brains having evolved in layers of distinct structures is not accepted in mainstream neuroscience.[167] Other criticism is of his methodology: Psychology professor Lisa Feldman Barrett, for example, considers his labelling of animal behaviours with human emotional descriptors as amounting to 'mental inference fallacies'. A brain circuit that activates during freezing behaviour, she says, only indicates exactly that: a freezing-behaviour circuit. To name the circuit 'fear' is to draw an inference about that action for which there is no evidence.[168]

Whether or not Panksepp's hypotheses stand the test of time, his approach brings into stark relief the strange disconnect that arises when brain science develops in parallel to the subjective, lived experience. How can you draw a conclusion about the brain of a person with anorexia without knowing how it feels to be that brain?

Indeed, the underlying tragedy to the traditional neurological view of the brain, Panksepp once said, was that it continued to treat the brain like a 'black box', where only stimulus going in and behaviour coming out were relevant to psychology. Even cognitive neuroscience, which finally acknowledged mental states, has only been willing to address them according to their physical correlates. But what behaviourism and cognitive neuroscience both left out, according to Panksepp, was human emotional experience: actual psychological states. The feeling of depression. The feeling of anxiety. The feeling of fearing food.

It is here that Panksepp found a natural ally in Mark Solms. The two brought their research together by saying, *If we pay attention to the way that a person describes how they* feel *when they are depressed* – that they lack motivation, desire, lose their appetite – *and we reasonably infer (both from the* DSM*'s acknowledgment that symptoms of depression and of grief can mirror each other and from the fact that our behavioural displays during depression are much like those during grief) that depression is profoundly connected to loss, we might be better placed to start researching depression by looking at the mammalian brain systems in place to generate this kind of feeling.*

What does all this mean, then, for humans in mental pain? First, it might give us insight into better-targeted pharmacological treatments. Taking depression as a case study, brain scan data has supported Panksepp's hypothesis that the neural network active in mammals during acute social loss or separation is the same one active in humans experiencing sadness and its related social processes.[169] These attachment-driven systems are mediated by the production or cessation of the chemicals opioids, oxytocin and prolactin. As Panksepp put it: 'too much activity in this system [PANIC/GRIEF] leads to a depletion of the seeking urge, which is the number one system for enthusiasm to live and do things. And we think that chemistries that can diminish panic, as well as those that can elevate seeking, might be good targets for antidepressants.'[170]

Biological pharmacology, then, might see great advances if researchers move away from the scattershot approach that resulted in SSRI treatments and focus instead on how the chemicals behind the attachment-driven systems work. Opiates, after all, were one of the first antidepressants, used to cure 'melancholy' in the nineteenth century, prescribed until the 1950s when those less addictive medications were stumbled upon by Roland Kuhn in his schizophrenia wards. Buprenorphine, for example, a non-addictive morphine derivative, is currently being trialled among antidepressant-resistant patients with major depressive disorder.[171]

Second, it might offer scientific rigour to the talking cure. Solms has used Panksepp's hypothesis of brain structure to propose a model of the mind that supports a psychoanalytic approach to treating emotional disturbance. He uses Freudian language to do this but, armed with the clearer structural view of the working brain that Panksepp has offered, he changes the parameters of Freud's concepts. Freud, he says, was wrong that the 'id' is unconscious. The id represents, rather, the conscious feeling states Panksepp referred to as *primary processes*, in the subcortical region. These feeling states can be elaborated into memory and learning by the *secondary processes*, mainly in the upper limbic region, which are extensively unconscious processes, and which go on to influence our *tertiary process* thoughts and cognitions. It is the middle level of process that Solms sees as more equivalent to Freud's 'ego', in being the part of ourselves that transforms our internal feeling-states into representations, both in the form of memories and words.

The ego, according to Solms, involves not only those internal feeling-states turned into representations but also a process in which we construct a representation of our own body as an object in the world, which is essentially an abstraction.

Solms's construction of ego, then, being the largely unconscious process by which memory and learning become thoughts and cognitions, and establish this representation of our self as an object in the world, is vital to understanding how the task of psychoanalysis might work, if we take that task as being 'to bring repressed thinking to consciousness'.

Solms says it is possible that what Freud called 'repression' is a situation in which cognition of a personal experience is interrupted so that it is not processed episodically (into a sort of autobiographical memory of events) but associatively (as the internal affects triggered during the experience). As with all learning, the person then automatises the association, so that it becomes a mental-behavioural 'algorithm' regardless of whether it suits reality.

As Solms explains: 'The therapeutic task of psychoanalysis, then, would be to undo repressions (to allow the affective distress associated with the repressed situation to emerge) in order to enable the ... subject to properly master it, and generate episodic representations adequate to the task, so that it may then be legitimately automatized.'[172] In simple terms, to help a person come to recognise the emotional experiences lingering in them that colour how they experience the world, and in doing so to give them a chance to relinquish them.

And what of the emotional systems Panksepp proposed? How are they relevant? 'Primal emotions unfold in relation to individual lives,' Solms says. The analyst, then, perhaps must come to know the patient well enough to understand their personal language as an expression of their primal emotional systems, and work with them to relearn the experiences of their life by reconnecting them to more constructive conscious realities.

Panksepp and Solms and the neuropsychoanalysts had given me a *prima facie* case to take back to Joni. *Look! The evidence of ancient affect structures in the brain! The basis of memory formation! Freud was right!* I would stack the pages up and bind them and get them published, and I would serve it to her like a warrant.

And they had proposed one possible answer to my question about Frankenstein's monster: conscious life emerges from a system of internal valence – our intrinsic sense of attraction or aversion – inherited evolutionarily from our mammalian ancestors that tells us how we feel so that we can propagate and survive (a far trickier plot point for Mary Shelley than a bolt of electricity).

To the question of where in me lay the sorrow of fathers leaving, they offered the addendum of *the individual life*: that a primal emotional system in me, perhaps the PANIC/GRIEF system along with the SEEKING system, may have been set up to malfunction as a result of events in my life; or, that I responded to separation with mental-behavioural algorithms that were developed in response to early life experiences.

But I no longer wondered that. Everything I had learned from the neuropsychoanalysts came down to this: I am both.

All I saw now was how strange and unworkable it had been to live a life in which I had not been able to conceive of being body *and* mind. That I had been unable to embody my own desires. That I had entered motherhood fundamentally unintegrated, part of me still attached to my metaphorical mother. That I was only born, myself, a long time afterward, when I found the words.

EPILOGUE

We came back from Holland. How would I end this story? That became my next question. Was there an end?

Freud was right, elementally, about the struggle he constructed in the Oedipus complex. The push and pull of the baby against the others in their life. That the baby has a first love, in their first carer. That they must concede to reality and give up their wish to obliterate their rival, whether it is their father, their mother, another third party or simply the presence of a world that takes their first love from them in other ways. But that wasn't science.

My father had left us. I did not have him to push and pull against. Sylvia Plath wrote her eviscerating poem 'Daddy', in which she tells her father she has had to kill him, even though he has died. Was it about her father? The essayist Katie Roiphe argues no; it was about her mother, from whom she struggled to separate. Plath's father had died when she was eight, leaving her unable to leave her mother.[173]

Melanie Klein was right, too. We can only face reality, mourn, live well, if we can bring together the love and hate – the ambivalence – we feel into the single object to which it belongs. My mother was the mother who breastfed me to contentment, who loved me so much she would fly across the globe without notice to have me safe in a Belsize Park hotel, and the mother who threatened my autonomy. My father was the father who left me when I was nine months old, and he was the father who came back as best he could, who offered me eternal love in the form of never-ending kisses.

They were both.

Aaron was overseas when the marriage-equality vote results came through. *YES.* It was a resounding yes. I had gone over to watch it with Paul, and we hugged and rejoiced. Our phones beeped with messages of excitement. Paul showed me one that came through from Maxine: *Finally! There's going to be a wedding! Mazel tov!* It occurred to me that Maxine had given me a gift by never ceasing to love my father, and by forgiving him.

'I have a lot of guilt. I should have done more when you were growing up,' my father told me when we were walking near the lake in Holland. He was talking about our childhood with my former stepfather. We used to speak on the phone every day back then. But it was possible he was talking about everything. About leaving. That if he had stayed I would not have felt my mother's survival depended on me. My actual mother. My dreamed-of mother. I would have been able to concede to reality.

There was nothing I could think to say. He put his arm around me and we walked on.

I railed at Dr Parkes for what he had not done for me. For not giving me sympathy, for not prescribing me medication. For not being there in the breaks when the spider dreams returned and my throat closed up and I needed him most. I railed at him and all he stood in for.

The brain science had seemed intractable so often. I had only skirted the edges of it. Detractors, questions of testability, replicability, loomed around every corner of firm knowledge I gained.

I could use the language of Panksepp and Solms to understand myself in terms of primal emotions and memory processes. Or I could say that my life was better set out in stories or poems. None of which could be proven. I will find my way, in the end, I told myself, with a Greek myth, with an article about a poet, with a blank page.

When we returned from Holland I began to write this into a book. I had been writing it all along, in the notepads I carried with me every day. I had been writing it when I scribbled down what Maxine and Aaron said, and when I highlighted and flagged Freud and Winnicott. When I printed out research papers. I had things in folders like a lawyer making a case, as though that's what I was doing. But I was writing a book.

A cat followed me into Dr Parkes's waiting area and sat directly opposite me. I didn't know what to do and began to laugh. Would it follow me into the consulting room? Would Dr Parkes pick it up?

'His name is Noah,' Dr Parkes told me, on discovering both the cat and me waiting for him. We laughed. I realised I had not laughed with him before.

Maybe I could be a mother and a writer and myself.

I had a dream. I was pregnant again. This time I went to see a doctor who could relieve the pain I felt from my unstable pelvis. I couldn't believe I had suffered, immobile, through two pregnancies when there had been a way to stop the pain. The doctor had an unusual method. I had to look at words. Individual words on tiny slips of paper. The doctor told me the individual words would come together visually in a way that made sense in my brain. That the part of the brain that put words together, when working, stopped bodily pain.

My mother was in my cells; my father was in my cells. And then I was my own body, made of them and entirely new.

Ψ

Psychoanalyst Darian Leader, who went looking for scientific literature on Freud's concept of mourning, found very little. *What had happened to our interest in how we come to terms with loss?* he wondered. Then it occurred to him that there was in fact a huge body of work on mourning, and it was in literature itself. The creation of art might allow us to come to terms with the losses in our selves.[174]

Every memory we have is the act of writing a story: 'Human memories are reconstructed and malleable,' explains cognitive neuroscientist Bruce Hood in his book *The Self Illusion*. 'We are constantly integrating the here and now into our past.'[175]

It was what I had been doing with Dr Parkes all along, too. The writer Siri Hustvedt, who has both psychoanalysis and neuroscience as interests, writes of the experience of psychoanalysis: 'What happens in the room is guided by theory, but the world forged between patient and analyst is also an intuitive, unconsciously driven, rhythmic, emotional, and often ambiguous undertaking. This is why doing analysis is something like making art.'[176]

Reuben told me he never again wanted to go on holiday.

'I don't ever want to leave home,' he said, indignantly, unaware of how his words alarmed me.

I told Dr Parkes: 'I am frightened that I have given Reuben my anxiety. I've given him my inability to go to France.'

'Well,' Dr Parkes responded, 'if you have the ability to give him something, you have the ability to take it away.'

There was the hope of change now.

Experimental psychologist Frederic Bartlett showed in his studies in the 1930s that each person repeats a story they have been told differently, according to their own ways of remembering, the ways their thought patterns and mental associations are organised. The stories we tell, the way we know our experience, makes each of our brains utterly unique. 'Nothing in biology makes sense except in the light of its own history,' writes neurologist Steven Rose in his book *The 21st-Century Brain*.

'I can't see how my postnatal feelings can be understood as anything other than a response to dramatic physiological changes,' I had said to Dr Parkes one day, when I had been determined to convince him that he had not helped me at all. 'The maternal brain actually changes. It makes new synaptic connections in order to be more vigilant, in order to love.'

'Yes, and you are making new synaptic connections right now, here with me,' Dr Parkes had responded.

Unlike the heart, the lungs, the bones, a brain cannot be understood as a static organ. It changes with its history and with every present moment. Neurons connect and cells are born, and die. The lived experience can never be excised from it as long as it is alive.

I phoned Joni one night: 'I just read a pretty strong argument that psychoanalysis is not a pseudo-science. I can send it to you,' I told her.

'Yeah?' she answered. 'Sure. I'll bet it's about Karl Popper. His way of classifying science has limitations.'

'It is!' I told her. 'God. Is there anything you don't know?'

She laughed. 'Actually, I've started seeing a therapist again,' she said. 'Psychodynamic.'

'What?' I was stunned.

'Yeah, yeah.' I could hear she did not want my opinion on this turn of events. She went on: 'Anyway. Hey, do you remember the time that girl came up to me at school and said that Dad loved her more than he loved me? Do you remember how upset I was?'

One memory had somehow lodged in us both as though it was ours. Or perhaps the feeling had been real and the little girl imagined.

Ψ

'Am I the best nanna?' Maxine asked Reuben, the next summer.

She leaned in to the open car window and smothered his face with kisses.

Then she came to my side and clutched the windowsill. 'I wanted to be the best mother,' she said to me, softly.

'We all do,' I replied, putting my hand on hers. 'We all do.'

I was back again, back again, back again, in the unsightly pleather rocking chair with baby Reuben, in my own white cot with my mother climbing in beside me, on the bench, crying, waiting with newborn Noah for my script to be filled. I went back again, back again, back again, to the source.

At some point I stopped lying on the couch. I wanted to face Dr Parkes, to see him. I was ready to feel for him, to have him be a real person. I saw we were wearing the same colours: navy blue, pink, cream. I remembered that he did not keep a notebook in his hand, as I had come to believe. The intermittent scribbling of his pen was imagined.

I looked at his face, it felt, for the first time.

Ψ

Noah points at the moon. 'Our moon?' he asks.

I tell him it is.

'We go there?' he asks.

I rest my chin on his head, in his curls, feel a ripple of love for the smell of him, his sweetness. (*You learn each other's scent; mammalian attachment*, Gideon told me after Reuben was born. Chemical hypnotism.)

'No,' I say. 'Not without a rocket ship.'

He turns his mouth down, disappointed. I think about the mental shift it must take for him to know the moon is out there in space, not some mark on a sheet of sky. And then I think about how the sun is not a light, controlled by a switch in human hands, but a giant ball of burning gas. I acknowledge the provenance of nature; the luck of it all.

Now my mind does what it does, in its treachery: the sun could go. We would die. It would be sudden and I might not be with my children when it happened. How can I keep them close so we can die together? How can we never be apart?

But I know that if I do this none of us will live.

Acknowledgements

With gratitude to:

Gideon, Reuben and Noah, for your love. You are my world.

Maxine and Aaron, for giving me my life, and for giving me, in your intellects, passions and empathy, the tools with which to understand it.

Joni, for your brilliance and friendship, and extensive research assistance.

Paul, for loving me as your child.

My parents-in-law, for your support and for the sanctuary of your home, always, and my sister- and brothers-in-law for supporting me, despite this strange work of writing that I do. Also, all the grandparents for allowing me to carve out time to do the writing, by helping with care for the children over the years.

Dr Parkes, for everything.

The Buddhist therapist, for what you gave me.

Professor Mark Solms and Dr Samantha Brooks for your time and incredible insight.

Emily Nozipo Mtsolongo, for mothering me; and for her children, wherever you are now, I acknowledge with sadness the loss you endured.

Zaida Perry, Granny Bella, Granny Fay and Grandpa Harvey, for all the ways you made me.

All my dear friends who were there through parts of this story over the decades with the gift of your friendship (especially all my cherished friends from my Sydney days, and also Kate and

Ryan Morris, Nicole Ford and Matthew Bennett; and Michelle, *te remercier de m'avoir sauve*), and with special mention to those who helped me verbally or otherwise to nut out aspects of this book: Lee Kofman, Rose Michael, Natalie Book, Ali Barker, Aletha Wilkinson, Bel Moneypenny, Steven Amsterdam, Jo Case, Nicola Berkovic, Kate Stanton, Aviva Tuffield (who, to my delight, became my publisher mid-way through the process), Emma Morris, Emma Schwarcz, Jenny Valentish, Melanie Joosten, and Writers' Loungers Lorien Kaye, Mary-Ellen Jordan and Ginger Briggs.

Creative Victoria and the Australia Council for the support through grants to allow me to give this work the attention it required.

Alexandra Payne, for your passionate interest in this book, and for your authentic care and careful attendance to it, and to me as your author.

Nikki Lusk, for your exceptional editorial work, and for insight wielded with the lightest but most incisive touch.

The team at UQP, including Madonna Duffy, Vanessa Pellatt, Kate McCormack, Kylie Rathborne and Jean Smith. Aziza Kuypers for her thorough proofread.

Helen Garner, for the time and attention you gave to reading my work and supporting it, and for your encouragement as I went along.

Siri Hustvedt, for reading and engaging so strongly with my work.

Finally, agent extraordinaire Jane Novak for championing my work from the get-go, and for all your wise and excellent advice and support.

Resources and support in Australia

General mental health

Lifeline (a national charity providing 24-hour crisis support and suicide prevention services): 13 11 14

beyondblue Support Service (a government bipartisan charity organisation engaged in mental health support and research): 1300 22 4636 (24 hours/7 days a week)

Postnatal mental health

Postnatal Anxiety & Depression Australia (PANDA) National Helpline: 1300 726 306 (Mon to Fri, 9 am – 7.30 pm AEST)

The Winn Clinic Consultation and Referral service (a perinatal mental health consultation and referral service for mothers and fathers during pregnancy and early childhood, subsidised by the Australian Psychoanalytic Foundation): access the service via an online application form at thewinnclinic.net, or contact Sonia Wechsler: perinatal@thewinnclinic.net

For a list of public early parenting centres offering residential stays with sleep and settling programs that attend to maternal mental health, see:
raisingchildren.net.au/articles/sleep_settling_help_babies_toddlers.html

Finding a psychoanalytic psychotherapist

The Australian Psychoanalytic Society:
psychoanalysis.asn.au/contact_find-an-analyst/

The Victorian Association of Psychoanalytic Psychotherapists: Referral service (03 9428 2303 to discuss your needs initially with a qualified psychotherapist) or visit: vapp.asn.au/

The Association for Psychoanalytic Psychotherapy WA:
appwa.org.au/appwa-psychoanalytic-psychotherapists

The NSW Institute of Psychoanalytic Psychotherapy:
nswipp.org/find-a-psychotherapist/

The Queensland Psychoanalytic Psychotherapy Association:
qppa.com.au/find-a-therapist/

New Zealand Institute of Psychoanalytic Psychotherapy:
psychotherapy.co.nz/therapists.html

Endnotes

1 Wulf Sachs, *Psychoanalysis: its meaning and practical applications*, Cassell & Co., London, 1934.
2 Sachs, p. 211.
3 Donald Woods Winnicott, 'Transitional objects and transitional phenomena', *International Journal of Psychoanalysis*, vol. 34, 1953, p. 93.
4 Marie Cardinal, *The Words to Say It* [*Les Mots Pour Le Dire*], trans. P Goodheart, Van-Vactor & Goodheart, Cambridge, MA, 1983 [1975], p. 248.
5 Donald Woods Winnicott, *Holding and Interpretation: fragment of an analysis*, Insitute of Psycho-Analysis, Karnac Books, London, 1989, p. 7.
6 Sigmund Freud, *Historical and Expository Works on Psychoanalysis*, Penguin, Harmondsworth, 1986, p. 284.
7 Neville Symington, *The Analytic Experience: lectures from the Tavistock*, St Martin's Press, New York, 1986, p. 16.
8 Patrick White, *Riders in the Chariot*, Vintage Classics, London, 1996 [1961], p. 57.
9 White, pp. 174–5.
10 Vivian Gornick, *Fierce Attachments: a memoir*, Simon & Schuster, New York, 1987, p. 189.
11 Robert M Kaplan, 'Treatment of homosexuality during apartheid: More investigation is needed into the shameful way homosexuality was treated', *British Medical Journal*, vol. 329, no. 7480, 2004, pp. 1415–16.
12 Donald Woods Winnicott, *Through Paediatrics to Psychoanalysis – collected papers*, Karnac Books, 1975, p. 195.
13 Wilfred Bion, *Learning from Experience*, Karnac Books, London, 1962.
14 Donald Woods Winnicott, *Playing and Reality*, Penguin Education, UK, 1982 [1971], p. 132.
15 Alice Miller, *The Drama of the Gifted Child: the search for the true self*, rev. ed., Basic Books, New York, 1997, p. 27.
16 Donald Woods Winnicott, 'Metapsychological and clinical aspects of

regression within the psycho-analytical set-up', *International Journal of Psychoanalysis*, vol. 36, 1955, p. 21.

17 Luce Irigaray, 'And the one doesn't stir without the other', trans. Hélène Vivienne Wenzel, *Signs: Journal of Women in Culture and Society*, vol. 7, no. 1, Autumn 1981, pp. 60–7.

18 Adrienne Rich, *Of Woman Born: motherhood as experience and institution*, Norton, New York, 1976, p. 236.

19 Nini Herman, *My Kleinian Home: a journey through four psychotherapies*, Quartet Books, London, 1985, p. 3.

20 Herman, p. 2.

21 Sigmund Freud, 'The question of lay analysis', in James Strachey (ed.), *Standard Edition of the Complete Psychological Works of Sigmund Freud* ('*SE*'), Hogarth Press, London, 1959, vol. XX, p. 252.

22 *Diagnostic and Statistical Manual of Mental Disorders*, fourth ed., American Psychiatric Association, 1994, pp. 186–7.

23 Gerald N Grob, 'Origins of *DSM-I*: of setting appearance and reality', *American Journal of Psychiatry*, vol. 148, 1991, pp. 421–31.

24 Shadia Kawa and James Giordano, 'A brief historicity of the *Diagnostic and Statistical Manual of Mental Disorders*: issues and implications for the future of psychiatric canon and practice', *Philosophy, Ethics, and Humanities in Medicine*, vol. 7, no. 2, 2012.

25 Judy Woodruff, 'What DSM-5, updated mental health "bible", means for diagnosing patients', *PBS News Hour*, 20 May 2013, pbs.org/newshour/bb/health-jan-june13-diagnosis_05-20/.

26 Pam Belluck and Benedict Carey, 'Psychiatry's guide is out of touch with science, experts say', *The New York Times*, 6 May 2013, nytimes.com/2013/05/07/health/psychiatrys-new-guide-falls-short-experts-say.html.

27 Sara Reardon, 'US mental-health agency's push for basic research has slashed support for clinical trials', *Nature*, 13 June 2017, nature.com/news/us-mental-health-agency-s-push-for-basic-research-has-slashed-support-for-clinical-trials-1.22145.

28 Peter Tyrer, 'A comparison of *DSM* and *ICD* classifications of mental disorder', *Advances in Psychiatric Treatment*, vol. 20, no. 4, July 2014, pp. 280–5.

29 Peter J Cooper and Lynne Murray, 'Course and recurrence of postnatal depression: evidence for the specificity of the diagnostic concept', *British Journal of Psychiatry*, 1995, vol. 166, no. 2, February 1995, pp. 191–5.

30 *The Penguin Freud Reader*, introduction by Adam Phillips, Penguin, London, 2006, p. 187.

31 Marion Milner, *A Life of One's Own*, Routledge, London, 2011, p. 158.

32 Letter from Freud to Eduard Silberstein, 9 September 1875, Freud Collection, D2, Library of Congress, as quoted in Peter Gay, *Freud: a life for our time*, Papermac, London, 1988, p. 26; Gay quote from p. 31 of the same.

33 Gay, p. xv.

34 Sigmund Freud, in *The Origins of Psychoanalysis: letters to Wilhelm Fliess, drafts and notes*, trans. Eric Mosbacher and James Strachey, Basic Books, New York, 1954, p. 137.

35 Sigmund Freud, *New Introductory Lectures on Psycho-analysis*, Hogarth Press, London, 1933.

36 Sigmund Freud and Josef Breuer, *Studies on Hysteria*, The Pelican Freud Library, vol. 3, Penguin Books, London, 1974, p. 272.

37 Ernest Jones, *The Life and Work of Sigmund Freud*, vol. 1, *The Formative Years and the Great Discoveries, 1856–1900*, Basic Books, New York, 1953, p. 29.

38 Sigmund Freud, 'Delusions and dreams in Jensen's *Gradiva*', *SE*, vol. IX, p. 7, quoted in Gay, p. 4.

39 Gay, p. 46, taken from Freud to Lothar Bickel, 28 June 1931. Typescript copy by permission of Sigmund Freud Copyrights, Wivenhoe.

40 Gay, p. 56.

41 Sigmund Freud, in *The Complete Letters of Sigmund Freud to Wilhelm Fliess, 1887–1904*, ed. and trans. Jeffrey Moussaieff Masson, Harvard University Press, Cambridge, MA, 1985, p. 184.

42 Gay, p. 58.

43 Janet Malcolm, *Psychoanalysis: the impossible profession*, Picador, London, 1982, p. 26.

44 Sigmund Freud, 'Studies on hysteria', *SE*, vol. II, p. 160.

45 Susanna Rustin, 'Adam Phillips: a life in writing', *The Guardian*, 2 June 2012, theguardian.com/books/2012/jun/01/adam-phillips-life-in-writing.

46 From Robert Reynolds, 'The inner and outer world of queer life', in Joy Damousi and Robert Reynolds (eds), *History on the Couch: essays in history and psychoanalysis*, Melbourne University Press, 2003, p. 48.

47 Herman, p. 2.

48 Donald Woods Winnicott, quoted in Josephine Klein, *Our Need for Others and Its Roots in Infancy*, Greener Books, London, 1994, p. 241.

49 Donald Woods Winnicott, 'The maturational processes and the facilitating environment: studies in the theory of emotional development', *The International Psycho-Analytical Library*, vol. 64, Hogarth Press and the Institute of Psycho-Analysis, London, 1965, p. 145.

50 Malcolm, p. 20.

51 Peter Gay speaking in *Young Dr Freud*, a film by David Grubin, produced by David Grubin Productions in association with PBS and Devillier Donegan Enterprises, 2002, pbs.org/youngdrfreud/pages/perspectives_women.htm.
52 Janet Sayers, *Mothering Psychoanalysis*, Penguin Books, London, 1991, p. 3.
53 Jonathan Lear, 'The shrink is in', *New Republic*, vol. 213, no. 26, 25 December 1995, pp. 18–25.
54 Sigmund Freud, 'On beginning the treatment', in *SE*, vol. XII, p. 127.
55 Sigmund Freud, 'An autobiographical study', in *SE*, vol. XX, p. 17.
56 Sigmund Freud, Preface to the translation of Bernheim's *On Suggestion*, quoted in Gay, p. 52.
57 Gay, p. 49.
58 Jon Stone et al., 'The "disappearance" of hysteria: historical mystery or illusion?' *Journal of the Royal Society of Medicine*. vol. 101, no. 1, January 2008, pp. 12–18.
59 Suzanne O'Sullivan, *It's All in Your Head: stories from the frontline of psychosomatic illness*, Vintage, London, 2016, p. 9.
60 Mary Shelley, *Frankenstein*, Modern Publishing Group, Australia, 1993 [1818], p. 40.
61 Susannah Cahalan, *Brain on Fire: my month of madness*, Simon & Schuster, New York, 2012, p. 9.
62 Hilary Rose and Steven Rose, *Genes, Cells and Brains: the Promethean promises of the new biology*, Verso, London, 2012, p. 253.
63 Joseph Fuhrmann, *Rasputin: the untold story*, John Wiley & Sons, Melbourne, 2012.
64 Mark Solms, 'Putting the psyche into neuropsychology', *The Psychologist*, vol. 19, September 2006, pp. 538–9, thepsychologist.bps.org.uk/volume-19/edition-9/special-issue-putting-psyche-neuropsychology.
65 Mark Solms, *The Feeling Brain: selected papers on neuropsychoanalysis*, Karnac Books, London, 2015.
66 Solms, *The Feeling Brain*, p. 3.
67 Jim Carrier, 'Lobotomies were once used to treat this gut disease, part of a shameful medical history', STAT, 12 June 2018, statnews.com/2018/06/12/lobotomy-ulcerative-colitis-shameful-medical-history/.
68 Symington, *The Analytic Experience*, p. 112.
69 Podcast, 'In writing: Adam Phillips in conversation with Josh Cohen', Freud Museum, London, 29 June 2017.
70 Wilfred Bion, *A Memoir of the Future*, Karnac Books, London, 1990, p. 578.

71 Wilfred Bion, *Cogitations*, Karnac Books, London, 1991, p. 377.
72 Malcolm, p. 144.
73 Carl R Rogers, *On Becoming a Person*, 1961, Houghton Mifflin, Boston, MA, p. 201.
74 Neville Symington, *A Healing Conversation*, Karnac Books, London, 2006, pp. 17, 19.
75 Elyn R Saks, *The Centre Cannot Hold: my journey through madness*, Kindle edition, Hachette, Sydney, 2007.
76 Sigmund Freud, 'The question of lay analysis', *SE*, vol. XX, p. 256.
77 Jonathan Shedler, 'The efficacy of psychodynamic psychotherapy', *American Psychologist*, vol. 65, no. 2, February–March 2010, pp. 98–109.
78 Podcast, 'In writing: Adam Phillips in conversation with Josh Cohen'.
79 Horst Kächele (ed.), *An Open Door Review of Outcome and Process Studies in Psychoanalysis*, third edn., International Psychoanalytic Association, London, 2015, p. 42.
80 Lane Strathearn, Peter Fonagy, Janet Amico and P Read Montague, 'Adult Attachment Predicts Maternal Brain and Oxytocin Response to Infant Cues', *Neuropsychopharmacology*, vol. 34, 2009, pp. 2655–66.
81 Peter Fonagy, in *An Open Door Review*, p. 59.
82 Eric R Kandel, 'Biology and the future of psychoanalysis: a new intellectual framework for psychiatry revisited,' *American Journal of Psychiatry*, vol. 156, no. 4, April 1999, p. 507.
83 Quoted from Francesca Ortu, 'Psychoanalysis and empirical research', *Rivista di Psicologia Clinica*, no. 1, 2007, p. 35.
84 Otto Kernberg, 'The pressing need to increase research in and on psychoanalysis', *International Journal of Psychoanalysis*, vol. 87, August 2006, p. 919.
85 Susan Sontag, *Illness as Metaphor*, Farrar, Straus & Giroux, New York, 1978, p. 5.
86 Bion, *Learning from Experience*, p. 99.
87 Andrea Hay, 'The Cape Town Child Guidance Clinic: an historical analysis, 1935–1971', unpublished thesis, University of Cape Town, 1990.
88 Thomas Szasz, *The Ethics of Psychoanalysis*, Syracuse University Press, New York, 1965, p. 182.
89 My thanks to the paper 'The analyst in the pharmacy' for a thorough outline of these arguments: Deborah Serani, *Journal of Contemporary Psychotherapy*, vol. 32, no. 2–3, September 2002, pp. 229–41.
90 Saks, loc. 3072.
91 Daniel Brass, 'Modelling containment in *Where the Wild Things Are* and *Outside Over There*', *Australasian Journal of Psychotherapy*, vol. 35, no. 1, 2017, p. 34.

92 E Molyneaux et al., 'Antidepressant treatment for postnatal depression', *The Cochrane Database of Systematic Reviews*, vol. 9, 11 September 2014.
93 V Sharma and C Sommerdyk, 'Are antidepressants effective in the treatment of postpartum depression? A systematic review', *The Primary Care Companion for CNS Disorders*, vol. 15, no. 6, 21 November 2013.
94 Diabetes Australia, 'More than 100,000 Australians have developed diabetes in the past year', diabetesaustralia.com.au/diabetes-in-australia.
95 Deloitte, *The Cost of Perinatal Depression in Australia*, 23 October 2012, www2.deloitte.com/au/en/pages/economics/articles/perinatal-depression-australia-cost.html.
96 beyondblue, clinical practice guidelines, 2011, beyondblue.org.au/health-professionals/clinical-practice-guidelines.
97 'Mental health care in the perinatal period', Australian Clinical Practice Guideline, October 2017, Centre of Perinatal Excellence, cope.org.au/wp-content/.../03/National-Perinatal-Mental-Health-Guideline-Final.pdf.
98 Mariana Angoa-Pérez et al., 'Mice genetically depleted of brain serotonin do not display a depression-like behavioral phenotype', *ACS Chemical Neuroscience*, vol. 5, no. 10, 2014, pp. 908–19.
99 Erick H Turner et al., 'Selective publication of antidepressant trials and its influence on apparent efficacy', *New England Journal of Medicine*, vol. 358, 2008, pp. 252–60.
100 I Kirsch et al., 'Initial severity and antidepressant benefits: a meta-analysis of data submitted to the Food and Drug Administration', *PLoS Medicine*, vol. 5, no. 2, February 2008.
101 F Hieronymus et al., 'Efficacy of selective serotonin reuptake inhibitors in the absence of side effects: a mega-analysis of citalopram and paroxetine in adult depression', *Molecular Psychiatry*, advance online publication, 25 July 2017.
102 Deborah Brauser, 'Final word? Antidepressants "do work"', *Medscape*, 29 August 2017.
103 Andrea Cipriani et al., 'Comparative efficacy and acceptability of 21 antidepressant drugs for the acute treatment of adults with major depressive disorder: a systematic review and network meta-analysis', *The Lancet*, published online, 21 February 2018.
104 Rose and Rose, p. 259.
105 David Healy, 'Serotonin and depression: the marketing of a myth', *British Medical Journal*, vol. 350, editorial, 21 April 2015.
106 Carmen P McLean, et al., 'Gender differences in anxiety disorders: prevalence, course of illness, comorbidity and burden of illness', *Journal of Psychiatric Research*, vol. 45, no. 8, August 2011, pp. 1027–35.

107 B Dell'Osso et al., 'Serotonin norepinephrine reuptake inhibitors (SNRIs) in anxiety disorders: a comprehensive review of their clinical efficacy', *Human Psychopharmacology*, vol. 25, no. 1, January 2010, pp. 17–29.
108 Rose and Rose, p. 254.
109 C Hazan and P Shaver, 'Romantic love conceptualised as an attachment process', *Journal of Personality and Social Psychology*, vol. 52, March 1987, pp. 511–24.
110 N Séjourné et al., 'Intergenerational transmission of postpartum depression', *Journal of Reproductive and Infant Psychology*, vol. 29, no. 2, 2011, pp. 115–24.
111 Miller, p. 7 (emphasis in original).
112 Maya Sela, 'The trauma of a gifted child whose mother was Alice Miller', *Haaretz*, 12 July 2014, haaretz.com/jewish/books/.premium-1.604326.
113 Miller, pp. 2, 10.
114 DF Simola et al., 'Epigenetic (re)programming of caste-specific behavior in the ant *Camponotus floridanus*', *Science*, vol. 351, no. 6268, January 2016.
115 Siddhartha Mukherjee, 'Same but different', *The New Yorker*, 2 May 2016, newyorker.com/magazine/2016/05/02/breakthroughs-in-epigenetics.
116 FA Champagne and JP Curley, 'Maternal regulation of estrogen receptor alpha methylation', *Current Opinion in Pharmacology*, vol. 8, no. 6, December 2008, pp. 735–9.
117 Lizzie Buchen, 'Neuroscience: in their nurture', *Nature*, vol. 467, 8 September 2010, pp. 146–8, nature.com/news/2010/100908/full/467146a.html.
118 Rachel Yehuda, et al., 'Influences of maternal and paternal PTSD on epigenetic regulation of the glucocorticoid receptor gene in Holocaust survivor offspring', *American Journal of Psychiatry*, vol. 171, no. 8, August 2014, pp. 872–80.
119 Josie Glausiusz, 'Doubts arising about claimed epigenetics of Holocaust trauma', *Haaretz*, 30 April 2017, haaretz.com/science-and-health/.premium-1.786465.
120 Tiago Castro e Couto et al., 'Postpartum depression: A systematic review of the genetics involved', *World Journal of Psychiatry*, vol. 5, no. 1, 22 March 2015, pp. 103–11.
121 Lisa S Segre and Wendy N Davis, 'Postpartum depression and perinatal mood disorders in the *DSM*', Postpartum Support International, 2013, postpartum.net/wp-content/uploads/2014/11/DSM-5-Summary-PSI.pdf.

122 Marie-Paule Austin et al., 'Depressive and anxiety disorders in the postpartum period: how prevalent are they and can we improve their detection?' *Archives of Women's Mental Health*, vol. 13, no. 5, 2010, pp. 395–401; beyondblue, 'Clinical practice guidelines for depression and related disorders – anxiety, bipolar disorder and puerperal psychosis – in the perinatal period', 2011.

123 A Viktorin et al., 'Heritability of perinatal depression and genetic overlap with nonperinatal depression', *American Journal of Psychiatry*, vol. 173, no. 2, 1 February 2016, pp. 158–65.

124 TC Eley, 'A twin study of anxiety-related behaviours in pre-school children', *Journal of Child Psychology and Psychiatry*, vol. 44, no. 7, October 2003, pp. 945–60.

125 Sigmund Freud, 'Mourning and melancholia', *SE*, vol. XIV, pp. 237–58.

126 Pilyung Kim, 'Human maternal brain plasticity: adaptation to parenting', *New Directions for Child and Adolescent Development*, vol. 153, 2016, pp. 47–58.

127 Pearson, Lightman and Evans, 2009; Raz, 2014; Roos et al., 2011, all cited in Kim, p. 49.

128 Kim and Bianco, 2014; Segre et al., 2007, all cited in Kim, p. 54.

129 S Levine et al., 'Behavioral and hormonal responses to separation in infant rhesus monkeys and mothers', *Behavioral Neuroscience*, vol. 99, no. 3, 1 June 1985, pp. 399–410.

130 V Hendrick et al., 'Hormonal changes in the postpartum and implications for postpartum depression', *Psychosomatics*, vol. 39, no. 2, March–April 1998, pp. 93–101.

131 M Bloch et al., 'Effects of gonadal steroids in women with a history of postpartum depression', *American Journal of Psychiatry*, vol. 157, no. 6, June 2000, pp. 924–30.

132 CE Schiller et al., 'The role of reproductive hormones in postpartum depression', *CNS Spectrums*, vol. 20, no. 1, February 2015, pp. 48–59.

133 Interview with Eric Kandel, *Spiegel Online*, 11 October 2012, spiegel.de/international/zeitgeist/interview-with-eric-kandel-psychoanalysis-art-and-biology-come-together-a-859702.html.

134 John M Harlow, 'Recovery from the passage of an iron bar through the head', Massachusetts Medical Society, 1868.

135 Mark Solms, 'What is a mind?' FutureLearning course, University of Cape Town, 2015.

136 Casey Schwartz, 'When Freud meets fMRI', *The Atlantic*, 25 August 2015, theatlantic.com/health/archive/2015/08/neuroscience-psychoanalysis-casey-schwartz-mind-fields/401999/.

137 Solms, *The Feeling Brain*, pp. 41–2.

138 Solms, *The Feeling Brain*, p. 68.

139 Solms, *The Feeling Brain*, p. 70.
140 Mark Solms, 'An example of neuro-psychoanalytic research: Korsakoff's syndrome', *European Journal of Psychoanalysis*, vol. 14, Winter–Spring 2002.
141 ibid.
142 Solms, *The Feeling Brain*, pp. 53–72.
143 Solms, *The Feeling Brain*, p. 82.
144 Solms, *The Feeling Brain*, p. 85.
145 Solms, 'An example of neuro-psychoanalytic research'.
146 JA Hobson and RW McCarley, 'The brain as a dream state generator: an activation-synthesis hypothesis of the dream process', *American Journal of Psychiatry*, vol. 134, no. 12, December 1977, pp. 1335–48.
147 Solms, *The Feeling Brain*, p. 130.
148 Mark Solms and Jaak Panksepp, 'Why depression feels bad', *Advances in Consciousness Research*, vol. 79, 2010, pp. 169–78.
149 G William Domhoff, 'Why did empirical dream researchers reject Freud? A critique of historical claims by Mark Solms', *Dreaming*, vol. 14, no. 1, March 2004, pp. 3–17.
150 J Allan Hobson, 'Freud returns? Like a bad dream', *Scientific American*, 1 April 2006, scientificamerican.com/article/counterpoint/.
151 Marshall Edelson, *Hypothesis and Evidence in Psychoanalysis*, University of Chicago Press, 1985, p. 110.
152 Rachel B Blass and Zvi Carmeli, 'The case against neuropsychoanalysis', *International Journal of Psychoanalysis*, vol. 88, 2007, p. 35.
153 ibid.
154 Sigmund Freud, 'Two principles of mental functioning', in *SE*, vol. XII, p. 225.
155 Blass and Carmeli, p. 36.
156 Yoram Yovell et al., 'The case for neuropsychoanalysis: why a dialogue with neuroscience is necessary but not sufficient for psychoanalysis', *International Journal of Psychoanalysis*, vol. 96, no. 6, December 2015, pp. 1515–53.
157 Eric R Kandel, 'Biology and the future of psychoanalysis: a new intellectual framework for psychiatry revisited', *American Journal of Psychiatry*, vol. 156, no. 4, April 1999, p. 507.
158 Pamela Weintraub, 'Jaak Panksepp pinned down humanity's 7 primal emotions', *Discover*, 31 May 2012, discovermagazine.com/2012/may/11-jaak-panksepp-rat-tickler-found-humans-7-primal-emotions.
159 Jaak Panksepp, *Affective Neuroscience: the foundations of human and animal emotions*, Oxford University Press, 2004, p. 167.
160 Solms, *The Feeling Brain*, p. 102.
161 Brian Johnson and Daniela Flores Mosri, 'The neuropsychoanalytic

approach: using neuroscience as the basic science of psychoanalysis', *Frontiers in Psychology*, vol. 7, no. 1459, 13 October 2016.

162 Weintraub.

163 Wilder Penfield and Herbert Jasper, *Epilepsy and the Functional Anatomy of the Human Brain*, Little and Brown, Oxford, 1954.

164 Antonio Damasio, *Descartes' Error*, Penguin, New York, 1994.

165 Weintraub.

166 Author correspondence with Samantha Brooks, 28 April 2016.

167 Suzana Herculano-Houzel goes into this in her 2016 book *The Human Advantage: a new understanding of how our brain became remarkable*, MIT Press, Cambridge, MA, 2016.

168 Lisa Feldman Barrett, *How Emotions Are Made: the secret life of the brain*, Houghton Mifflin Harcourt, Boston, MA, 2017, ch. 12.

169 Damasio et al., 'Subcortical and cortical brain activity during the feeling of self-generated emotions', *Nature Neuroscience*, vol. 3, no. 10, October 2000, pp. 1049–56.

170 'The emotional foundation of mind: Dr Jaak Panksepp – a Dr Dave Van Nuys interview', *The Neuropsychotherapist*, vol. 2, July–September 2013, p. 98.

171 'Alkermes Announces Initiation of FORWARD-3 and FORWARD-4 Efficacy Studies in Pivotal Program for ALKS 5461 for Treatment of Major Depressive Disorder', press release, Alkermes, phx.corporate-ir.net/phoenix.zhtml?c=92211&p=irol-newsArticle&ID=1938539.

172 Solms, *The Feeling Brain*, p. 176.

173 Katie Roiphe, '"Daddy" Is Mommy', *Slate*, 11 February 2013, slate.com/articles/double_x/roiphe/2013/02/sylvia_plath_s_poem_daddy_is_about_her_mother.html.

174 Darian Leader, *The New Black: mourning, melancholia and depression*, Penguin Books, London, 2008, p. 6.

175 Bruce Hood, *The Self Illusion: why there is no 'you' inside your head*, Constable & Robinson, London, 2012, p. 57.

176 Siri Hustvedt, *A Woman Looking at Men Looking at Women: essays on art, sex and the mind*, Sceptre, London, 2016, p. 120.